This information this book is not intended to be medical advice and should not be relied upon as a substitute for consulting with your physician. The information contained within may not address all possible actions, treatments or therapies, precautions, side-effects or interactions. All manners regarding your health require the supervision of a physician who is familiar with your medical needs. For more information please contact your physician.

Some of the Web site information in this book may change with time. The Web sites listed in this book were current as of September 22, 2012.

i

Dedication:

To my mentor, David L. Page, M.D., a giant among physicians and to my friend Michele Norris, without whose support this book would not have come to be. I thank my husband Mark S. Ross and my daughters Alexandra and Estrella for their patience and support.

Table of Contents

Preface: Landing in a foreign country

I am a pathologist. My job is to look through the microscope at the cells in tissue sections from patients' biopsies or surgeries. I read the notes in the medical record about why the patients have undergone a biopsy or surgery. Then it is my job to decide whether or not they have cancer or anything in the spectrum that exists between normal cells and cancer. I work with teams of surgeons, oncologists, and other pathologists in formulating treatment plans for patients. My job is to classify the cells that I see so that their diagnosis will fit into the best treatment plan.

Quite often, friends of mine will have a medical question. Someone close to one of them will have been given a diagnosis of cancer. As I listen to my friends, I feel as though they have been taken out of the world that they know and have been transported to another world where the language is supposed to be English, but everything is unfamiliar. For several years now, I have been a resource for them. This informal role has increased, until finally my very close friend Michele said, "You should write a book." And here I am.

There are many books on cancer. Why is this one different? This book is a *pocket guide*. I will not go into a lot of technical details such as the risks of cancer, how normal cells become cancer cells, or treatment for specific cancers. Treatment varies somewhat from hospital to hospital and tremendously from tumor to tumor. It also tends to change over time. Because of this, such a book would soon be out of date, and there are already books available that include details about risk factors and therapy.

Thus, this book was written to be something that you, as a patient or as someone acting in the role of caregiver or advocate to a patient, can easily carry around, and yet it still is substantive enough to have the basic information that will help you make decisions about the diagnosis and treatment of cancer. My goal is to empower you as a patient or caregiver in a short amount of time so you can join in a partnership with the doctor and take ownership of the treatment plan.

Chapter 1. What is cancer?

Terms discussed in this chapter (listed alphabetically)
Atypia
Borderline tumor or cancer (see also Chapter 6)
Distant metastasis
Dysplasia
Grade
In situ cancer
Invasive cancer
Isolated tumor cells
Micro-invasive cancer
Micrometastasis
Regional metastasis
Stage
Superficially invasive cancer

Getting started

This chapter is a "crash course" in cancer terminology. Even without the emotional overlay that comes with a diagnosis of cancer, the territory seems unfamiliar to patients and their caregivers because we doctors have developed a vocabulary and syntax of our own. We try to standardize our diagnoses and our evaluation of the patient in the same way that we standardize weight and time in our everyday life. In this first chapter, I will start with a brief description of the types of doctors involved in collecting the information required to make a treatment plan for your cancer. I will also introduce important terms that are used to describe cancer.

As a pathologist, my job is to look through a microscope and examine the cells in tissue from a patient's biopsy or surgery and diagnose them as normal, cancerous, or something in-between. Then I assess the measures agreed upon in the medical world and present them in the report.

More aggressive cancers need more aggressive treatment plans, and less aggressive cancers need less aggressive treatment plans. A cancer that either has been growing for a long time undetected or is very aggressive from the start may have spread to distant parts of the body by the time it is diagnosed. At this stage, this cancer may need yet another plan of treatment.

Standardized measures shape this kind of information when it is passed on to other members of the medical team. The advantage of using the standardized measures is that an oncologist or surgeon anywhere can read a pathology report, understand it, and put together a treatment plan for a patient. The downside is that our vocabulary has evolved to promote better communication between physicians, but it does not show consideration for how to convey this same information to the patient.

Anyone who has not previously been diagnosed with cancer may not be aware of the spectrum of cancerous conditions or the spectrum of accuracy with which they are now being diagnosed. This is like being given a map without a legend. At a time when a patient needs to gather information and make decisions, she might not even know the right questions to ask.

I will give you an overview of the process that doctors use to put together the map for your particular cancer treatment. I will tell you about important questions you need to ask to define the legend for your map. I have generalized these so that they can apply to any patient. In the end, I want you as the patient, or the caregiver, to be empowered to navigate your own journey through what seems mystifying at first, the world of cancer and its treatment.

A criticism that could be made of this book is that I do not address important issues of health insurance coverage in the United States. That is a yet another book. Also, when I talk about decision-making, I will try to describe an ideal patient—doctor relationship. I recognize that not all

2

such relationships are ideal, but I encourage each and every one of you who has cancer, or who is helping someone who has cancer, to strive for an ideal relationship with who for you is an ideal doctor.

Cancers that require aggressive treatment with invasive surgery and/or toxic chemotherapy and radiation will test the best of relationships, and the treatment plan may fail. From the beginning, you should assemble a team that cares in the best way for you, who are excellent in their specialty, with whom you have excellent communication, who can discuss their decision-making process with you in as much detail as you want, and with whom you can trust your life. **Always remember—you are the patient—and as such you have the right to ask questions and the right to change doctors.**

Who are my doctors?

Your treatment team is made up of several specialists. The **medical oncologist** is the doctor who gives you chemotherapy or other drugs. A **radiation oncologist** treats you with radiation. Your **surgeon** operates on you. Two specialists that you may not meet in person are the **radiologist** and the **pathologist**. Your radiologist interprets your imaging studies, such as x-rays, mammograms, ultrasounds, CT scans, and MRIs, to look for abnormalities that might be cancer.

Your pathologist interprets your laboratory tests and decides whether or not they show that you actually have cancer, and how aggressive it is. Your laboratory tests can involve blood tests; urine samples; body fluid drawn from a particular location such as your spinal fluid; or any piece of tissue removed as part of a small biopsy procedure or as part of a larger surgery. Your pathologist is a key figure in your team of specialists. You need to have a diagnosis of cancer that is made on the actual cancer cells in your body before you can be treated.

3

How does a pathologist decide that I have a malignant cancer?

Pathologists like myself look at cells from patient's biopsies and assign them a diagnosis based on how fast they are dividing, their size and shape, how they congregate, and how other types of cells next to them react to their presence. There is a continuum of abnormal states between normal and cancerous that we have separated into several categories.

The categories of diagnosis are *normal*, *atypical* (frisky), *dysplastic* (has a gang mentality), *in situ* (a gang that is contained within a certain location), *micro-invasive* or *superficially invasive* (a gang that is just barely starting to spread beyond its borders), or *invasive* (a gang that is capable of spreading away from its home base). Invasive cancer is considered *malignant*. Malignant tumors can invade and destroy local tissue, and they can spread to distant parts of the body.

What is the difference between *in situ* and invasive or malignant cancer?

In situ is Latin for "in its normal place." The most common cancers go through a series of states starting with dysplasia, and followed by an *in situ* cancer that is held back by a natural containment system called the basement membrane. Cancers need to be able to get into *blood vessels* or special drainage systems for fluid called *lymphatic channels* in order to be able to spread to other sites. While *in situ*, a cancer does not have access to blood vessels or lymphatic channels, and so it cannot travel to other sites.

But when cancer becomes invasive, it crosses the dividing line between *in situ* and malignant. Very literally, it chews through the basement membrane and can get access to blood vessels and lymphatic channels.

Very early invasion in which there is still almost no likelihood of spreading to distant sites is called micro-invasive. Superficially invasive is also an early state of invasion where there is only a small possibility that this cancer has spread outside of its native organ system. Invasive, when it has not been described as micro-invasive or superficially invasive, means that the cancer is well beyond the basement membrane. It is capable of spreading out, not only locally in its native organ system, but also by appearing in or *metastasizing* to distant sites in the body. *In situ* cancer cannot metastasize. Invasive or malignant cancer *can* metastasize.

Do all cancers have an *in situ* stage?

With the *in situ* state, we begin to think of these cells as having become a cancer, although there is a big difference between *in situ* and invasive or malignant cancer as was pointed out in the preceding answer. Whether or not there is an *in situ* stage is actually a function of the type of cell that becomes the cancer.

A simple rule to follow is that cancers whose medical name includes *carcinoma* will have an *in situ* stage. Melanoma is a special case of a cancer that is not a carcinoma and yet has an *in situ* stage before it becomes malignant. Brain cancer, leukemia, lymphoma, and cancers whose medical name ends in *sarcoma* do not have an *in situ* state, but they do have a malignant state. These cancers sometimes have an intermediate state between benign (not cancer) and malignant that is called *borderline*. Borderline tumors will be discussed in more detail in Chapter 6.

What does metastasizing mean?

When we say that a cancer is capable of *metastasizing,* we mean that the cancer is capable of spreading to distant sites. By distant sites, I mean other organ systems or body sites. The cancer in the original site or organ in which it developed is called the *primary cancer,* commonly referred to as the *primary*. If it has spread to another site, then this colony of foreign cancer cells is called a *metastasis* (plural is *metastases*). For a metastasis to occur, a single cancer cell or a cluster of cancer cells must be able to break away from the primary cancer, implant themselves in another site, and grow there. A metastasis is usually a sign of a more aggressive or a more advanced cancer that will need more aggressive treatment.

Do all cancers have to be capable of metastasizing to be considered malignant?

With a few exceptions, a cancer is considered malignant when it is capable of metastasizing. Brain cancer is an important exception. This cancer does not have to be capable of metastasizing to be considered malignant. This is because it is growing in a critical organ system. The simple fact is that if it is invasive and fingering out into the normal brain tissue around it, then it is difficult to remove surgically and it is a very serious disease.

Are metastases always a sign of a more advanced cancer?

In mot cancers this is true, but not for all cancers. Metastases are not considered important in discussing lymphoma and leukemia. By itself, the ability to metastasize is not a sign of a more advanced cancer since these cancers start out in several sites. There can be some special considerations though for lymphoma and leukemia, such as whether there is brain involvement or not.

Are all metastases equal as a sign of aggressiveness?

Not all metastases are considered equal. They are rated according to whether they are regional or distant. *Regional metastases* are bits of tumor that have broken off and implanted in a nearby site that is not the same place that the primary cancer developed in. For example, metastases to local lymph nodes are regional metastases. If the cancer cells travel to another organ system or a site further away in the body, implant themselves, and continue to grow, then this is called a *distant metastasis*. Regional metastases are in locations that are easier for the primary tumor to reach. They might be the nearest lymph nodes, which act like a filter to catch bits of tissue breaking off. Distant metastases are in locations that are more difficult for the primary tumor to reach. A distant metastasis is a more serious sign than a regional metastasis.

For some cancers, we distinguish between a few *isolated tumor cells* in a lymph node, a small cluster of cells only a few millimeters in size and called a *micrometastasis*, and a larger cluster of tumor cells that indicates that there is an established regional metastasis. For example, in breast cancer, isolated tumor cells in a lymph node do not mean that such cancer cells can actually survive in a foreign territory. Thus they are not used to determine your stage. Your doctor may want to take into account that their presence means that this cancer is able to get into the lymphatic channels and travel around, but such isolated tumor cells are not counted as a metastasis. Similarly, micrometastases, depending on your tumor type, may not impact your treatment plan or outcome.

Is metastasizing the only way that cancer can spread to another organ?

No, a cancer can grow directly into another organ if it originates in a body site where several organs are close to one another. The cancer may spread from one organ to the next just by growing into the adjacent organ system. This is called *contiguous* involvement of other organs. In this case, cancers don't have to break off and enter a blood vessel or lymphatic channel to spread to other sites. Colon cancer may spread to the bladder, or stomach cancers may spread to the colon, by contiguous spread.

Will I only be treated if my cancer is invasive or malignant?

No, in many cases you will also be treated if you have *in situ* cancer, a borderline tumor, and in some cases, dysplasia. Whether you are treated depends upon the risk

7

of an invasive or malignant cancer developing from either the dysplasia, the borderline tumor, or the *in situ* cancer. This constitutes the basis for early treatment to prevent the development of malignant cancer.

The treatment plan, in this case, is usually removal, either by or some form of ablation (killing of the cells). Ablation commonly uses laser beams to burn the cells or cryotherapy to freeze the cells. Chemoprevention, using drugs with a low side-effect profile, is also used as a therapy. If you have a diagnosis of mild dysplasia, sometimes called atypia, you will generally be offered increased surveillance to watch for the possible development of a cancer. However, you should not worry about possible metastases, because, in this case of course, your cancer was not invasive.

Are all cancers equally bad?

No, cancers range from types that will probably have no effect on how long you live to cancers that are very aggressive. Instances of cancer are classified by a pathologist to indicate how they will behave. In general, pathologists classify cancers first, according to their primary organ site; second, according to what type of cell the cancer cell originated from; and third, by subtypes that can be recognized and distinguished, and that imply different behaviors of the cells.

Then, at the subtype level, the cancer is assigned a grade to indicate how aggressive it can be expected to behave. *Grade* is thus a measure how severely abnormal the cells are. Over years of studying cancer under the microscope, pathologists have agreed on grading systems that correlate with how aggressively the cancer cells will behave. Different cancer types will have different grading systems, which are fine-tuned to measure the cancer's aggressiveness.

Grade is such a useful measure that it is also used to describe dysplastic cells and *in situ* cancer. The higher the grade, the more likely the cells are to advance to the next level. For lung and breast cancer, grade is divided into three categories: low-grade or well-differentiated; intermediate grade or moderately differentiated and high grade or poorly differentiated. In colon cancer and in bladder cancer, only two grades are used, low and high.

In prostate cancer, the most common grading system is the Gleason grade, in which there are five grades. Grade 1 is the lowest and grade 5 is the highest. Prostate cancer also has something called the *Gleason score*. As a practical finding, prostate cancer often has multiple grades in the same patient; thus, the Gleason score is the sum of the two most prevalent grades. If there is only one grade present, then that grade is doubled. So a prostate cancer that is in all instances in a patient Gleason grade 3 will yield a Gleason score of 6. A case of prostate cancer with mostly Gleason grade 3 and some Gleason grade 4 will have a Gleason score of 7.

How is stage used to classify the spread of the cancer?

In addition to the primary organ, type, subtype, and grade of a cancer, the *stage* of the cancer at the time of diagnosis is a very important measure for determining how a patient will be treated. The stage is *a measure of how far this cancer has been able to grow or spread in the body.* For most cancers, stage is determined by a combination of: how big the primary tumor is or how deep it has grown within its primary organ system, whether it has spread regionally, either via metastases to local lymph nodes or by contiguous growth to nearby organs; and whether it has spread to distant sites.

In cancers in which local lymph nodes are important, the stage can be broken down into three parts.

- The *T stage* is a measure of the tumor size or how deep within a tissue a tumor has grown. For example, in breast cancer, tumor size is used. In colon cancer, the T stage is a measure of *how deep* into the wall of the colon the tumor has grown.

- The N stage is a measure of how many lymph nodes are involved.

- The M stage is a measurement of whether or not distant metastases are present.

For any one cancer type, there is a rule-set, an algorithm that combines the T, N, and M stages to yield an overall stage for the patient. The National Cancer Institute collects survival data for each stage for most cancers. Stage will be described again in Chapters 4 through 6 which discuss diagnosis and treatment.

Leukemia and lymphoma do not follow this staging system. More important with these cancers is whether or not there is brain involvement. Some doctors use a staging system for lymphoma that considers whether or not it is contained within one half of the body. For brain cancers, because spread to other parts of the body is not an issue, stage is not as important as the grade and exactly where the cancer is located.

What does my tumor type, grade, and stage have to do with my prognosis and treatment?

Tumor type, grade, and stage, with the exceptions described above, are critical to determining how a patient will be treated. Other factors to be taken into account are how healthy a patient is, how old he or she is, and the desires of that individual patient with respect to how aggressive a treatment he or she might be willing to undergo. This is addressed in more detail in Chapter 7.

Prognosis for a patient is measured by survival after 5 years from diagnosis (called 5-year overall survival) and by recurrences within 5 years (called 5-year recurrence-free survival). These data are continually recorded by cancer data registries. Every few years the National Cancer Institute recalculates the expected incidence rates and 5-year survival for cancer patients at large and publishes these updated statistics as the Surveillance Epidemiology and End Results (see the Web sites section at the end of this chapter). These statistics are broken down by cancer type, stage, gender, race, age, and state of residence. A descriptive summary of prognoses for different cancer types can be found at the American Cancer Society Web site included in the list of Web sites at the end of this chapter.

How accurate is my diagnosis?

Pathologists are charged with determining a diagnosis from a continuous spectrum of cell behaviors and placing it into one of the five categories ranging from normal to invasive as described above. In addition to interpreting the category that the disease should fall into, pathologists also convey just how sure they are of the diagnosis. I myself use terms such as

- "not diagnostic of" (meaning if you are suspicious something is there you need to investigate it further);

- "cannot exclude the possibility of" (meaning that there is something here that bothers me but it is not clear what it is—either it should be investigated further or you should keep a close eye on this patient);

- "suggestive of" (meaning, you should think about the possibility of this diagnosis and you should investigate further);

- "suspicious for" (meaning, it is not picture perfect, but I am worried about this possibility, and more tests or a re-biopsy is needed to make sure this is not cancer);

- "compatible with" (meaning that I cannot say with 100 percent accuracy but taken together with other things I know about the patient, this diagnosis would fit);

11

- "consistent with" (meaning that this diagnosis fits all of the data but the data don't exclude all other possibilities);

- "diagnostic of" (I am sure).

Not only is the disease on a continuum, but our sense of the accuracy with which we can diagnose something follows a continuum.

Web sites for cancer statistics

http://seer.cancer.gov/ The Surveillance Epidemiology and End Results published, by the National Cancer Institute. Select the "Cancer Statistics" tab (or go directly there by going to http://seer.cancer.gov/statistics). You can either select "Fast Stats" to access the statistics organized by organ site, ethnicity, gender, and other variables, or for more detailed information about the SEER statistics select "Cancer Statistics Review". By selecting the "Publications" tab, you can access the link to "Monographs" and select the latest "SEER Survival Monograph" for perusal.

Reports you should ask for from your doctor if you have been diagnosed with cancer

Pathology reports
Radiology reports

Chapter 2. Who gets cancer and why is family history important?

Terms discussed in this chapter (listed alphabetically)
Chemoprevention
Genetic susceptibility
Germline mutation
Prophylactic surgery
Prophylaxis
Somatic mutation
Surveillance
The Genetic Information Nondiscrimination Act of 2008

Who gets cancer?

Anybody can get cancer. There are fetal cancers, childhood cancers, and cancers of young adulthood. Certain cancers occur more commonly in males than in females; vice versa is true for certain other cancers. The most common cancers are more prevalent in the aging population, but not exclusively so. Lung, breast, colon, and prostate cancer also occur in young to middle-aged adults, but are rare in children. Ninety-five percent of lung cancer cases can be attributed to smoking. Embryonic rhabdomyosarcoma is an infrequent cancer. It predominantly affects children, and rarely young adults.

Do cancers run in families?

Cancer can run in families, or they can be sporadic. For example, nearly half of the cases of retinoblastoma, a childhood cancer of the retina, occur with a strong family history. These *familial cancers* occur because of an underlying genetic susceptibility caused by a mutation in a specific gene that is passed on from parent to child. In the case of retinoblastoma, this is the retinoblastoma, or Rb, gene. Patients with familial cancers will have a "strong family history" of that cancer. This means that several relatives over several generations have had that cancer.

A sporadic cancer is one that occurs randomly among individuals in the population, and there is no pattern in the patient's family tree that suggests a genetic susceptibility. A little more than half of the cases of retinoblastoma are sporadic. This means that this is the first time it has been diagnosed in your family tree.

What does genetic susceptibility mean?

A cancer cell will have some combination of genetic abnormalities. More than one genetic abnormality is required, but if you are born with one already, then you are partway to developing cancer. This is called *genetic susceptibility* and it means you could develop cancer at a younger age than usual. If you inherited the genetic abnormality, then testing for this abnormality can be used to understand how susceptible you might be to that cancer.

Are all genetic abnormalities inherited, so that once I have cancer, by virtue of that, my children will be susceptible?

No, not all genetic abnormalities are inherited, but some are. Genetic abnormalities can be *germline* or *somatic*. *Germline* means that your children can inherit the genetic tendency to develop cancer. *Somatic* means that the tissue that developed the cancer had an injury that damaged some of its genes. A somatic abnormality is only in that spot and will not affect your children. Examples of somatic abnormalities are the ones that occur from sun damage to the skin, which can cause skin cancer.

There is one more thing to add about germline genetic abnormalities, and that is whether they are *inherited* or *sporadic*. *Inherited* means that you inherited the genetic abnormality from one of your parents, so your siblings might also have that abnormality in addition to your children. A *sporadic* germline mutation occurs when the genes that define your germline are being prepared. This can be at any step in the development of the genes that are packaged in an egg or a sperm. You did not inherit this mutation, and your siblings won't be at risk, but you can pass the mutation on to your children.

What are some examples of cancers that can be inherited?

Of the four most common cancers in the United States today—lung, breast, colon, and prostate—most cases are not associated with a strong family history. Even so, there are germline mutations that give patients a high risk for developing some of these cancers. For example, patients with a mutation in the genes named BRCA1 or BRCA2 have a high risk of developing breast cancer. Patients with BRCA2 mutations also have a high risk of developing ovarian cancer. Both men and women with a mutation in a DNA mismatch repair gene, most frequently the genes MLH1 and MSH2, have a high risk of developing a gastrointestinal cancer, presenting predominantly as a colon cancer, which is referred to as Hereditary Non-Polyposis Colon Cancer. Women in these families have a higher risk than the average person of developing breast, ovarian or uterine cancer. This familial cancer occurrence has also been called *Lynch Syndrome*, and Dr Henry T. Lynch, who discovered the inheritance pattern.

How does environmental exposure cause cancer?

Any time that cells divide, even under normal conditions, they may acquire some mistake in the genetic code. In addition, environmental exposures cause genetic abnormalities that can accumulate to cause cancer. More recently, we have been learning about how environmental factors combine with germline genes to increase the risk of developing cancer.

In the case of lung cancer, we have known for several years that it has a strong association with smoking. Most cases of lung cancer occur in smokers, but most smokers do not develop lung cancer. As we continue to do research, we are discovering heritable factors that make it more likely for a smoker to develop lung cancer.

15

There was a recent report about the association of two *single nucleotide polymorphisms*, or SNPs (pronounced "snips"), with the development of lung cancer in some smokers. A SNP is a mutation in a single read-out of a gene—a single "typo" so to speak—that by itself does not have a noticeable effect on a person's health. However, if it occurs in a gene that inactivates toxins in the body, then that person will be more sensitive to the affects of that toxin. In the case of lung cancer, as of what we know now, SNPs in two different genes, together with a history of smoking, increase that person's risk for developing lung cancer. As a result, the inheritance pattern has not been obvious. The association of germline SNPs with cancer risk is a very exciting topic of research right now, but as yet there are no screening tests for these newly discovered SNPs.

What steps should I consider if I have a strong family history of cancer?

If you have a strong family history of cancer, or if someone closely related to you has a known germline mutation, then you should see a genetic counselor to learn about your personal risk of developing cancer. There is a Web site listed at the end of this chapter that has information on cancer centers that perform genetic counseling. There may be a test for a specific genetic abnormality that you can have performed. You should also discuss a surveillance plan with your doctor, which may mean more frequent screening tests for cancer. In addition to increased surveillance, there are also prophylaxis plans that people use to prevent cancer. This can be in the form of chemoprevention (taking medicine), or it can be prophylactic surgery.

What is prophylactic surgery?

Prophylactic surgery is the removal of the site or organ that is at risk. Examples of prophylactic surgery are the removal of your ovaries to prevent ovarian cancer, the removal of your breasts to prevent breast cancer, or the removal of your colon to prevent colon cancer. You should at least know what kind of prophylaxis is available to you if you have a strong family history, or a known mutation, that raises your cancer risk.

Prophylactic surgery is an extreme step, but it might also benefit you. Also remember that the choice is yours. You need to be informed as to how effective the prophylaxis plan is in preventing the cancer. For example, women who undergo prophylactic removal of the breast still have a small risk, because not all of the breast tissue is removed in a mastectomy. Depending on the patient's personal anatomy, a small amount near the shoulder usually remains, and it is not easily monitored by mammography.

Can the health insurance companies refuse to insure me because I have a genetic susceptibility?

Not after May 2009 they can't. On May 21, 2008, President Bush signed the Genetic Information Nondiscrimination Act (GINA) of 2008. This new federal law protects us from being discriminated against by health insurers and by employers because of our genetic make-up. The parts of the law that address health insurers are in effect as of May 2009, and those relating to employers are in effect as of November 2009. For more information, check the Genetic Discrimination Fact Sheet at the National Human Genome Research Institute (NHGRI) Web site.

Web sites for information about genetic testing

http://www.nsgc.org/ is a Web site maintained by the National Society of Genetic Counselors. They provide a link for finding a genetic counselor near you.

http://www.genome.gov/10002328#3 is a Web site maintained by the National Human Genome Research Institute (NHGRI). It has a fact sheet about the Genetic Information Nondiscrimination Act (GINA) of 2008

Web sites for information about genetic testing, continued

http://www.genome.gov is the web site for the home page of the National Human Genome Research Institute (NHGRI) Web site. It contains general information about the state of research into human genetics

---

Questions for your doctor if you have been diagnosed with cancer

Where can I get genetic counseling?

Are there genetic tests to consider for my cancer type? How accurate are these tests?

Can they detect all of the types of abnormalities in a particular gene that causes this cancer?

What can I do with this information?

Should my brothers and sisters be tested? Should my children be tested?

How can I make sure that my ability to get health insurance is protected by the Genetic Information Nondiscrimination Act?

How will my genetic susceptibility affect my ability to get life insurance?

Questions for your doctor if you are considering chemoprevention or prophylactic surgery

What are the chances I will develop cancer without prophylaxis?

Can I tolerate this surgery?

What are the side-effects?

What are the cosmetic effects?

Can I get reconstruction or a prosthetic?

Questions for your doctor if you are considering chemoprevention or prophylactic surgery, continued

Can I still get this cancer after prophylaxis? (This can happen when the tissue of the susceptible organ system cannot be completely removed.)

Do I need to continue to be monitored after prophylactic therapy?

How easy is it for a doctor to monitor me if I need it?

Is there a chemoprevention drug that can act against the types of cancers that I might get?

Chapter 3. How is cancer detected early?

Abbreviations and Terms discussed in this chapter
(listed alphabetically)

Abbreviations:
ACS American Cancer Society
CDC Centers for Disease Control and Prevention
NCI National Cancer Institute
Terms:
BIRADS
Colonoscopy
False negative
False positive
Mammography
PSA
Pap smear
Screening recommendations

What are screening tests?

Screening tests are designed for early detection of cancer. They can either look directly for cancer, such as a colonoscopy, or they can select out patients who are more likely to have cancer, such as the prostate specific antigen (PSA) blood test for risk of having prostate cancer. Cervical cancer screening by Pap smears (Papanicolaou test after Georgios Papnikolaou, also called Pap smear) is a great success story because it has reduced the burden of death due to cervical cancer in women since it was introduced in the 1950s.

How do I find out what the current screening recommendations are for me?

The American Cancer Society (ACS), the Centers for Disease Control and Prevention (CDC), and the National Cancer Institute (NCI) all maintain Web sites with current screening recommendations. The recommendations differ slightly at each site depending upon the cancer that is being screened for. When the recommendations differ, it is important for you to consider what is best for you as an individual. Your own personal screening schedule should be based on your personal risk and family history. It is a good idea to talk with your physician about cancer screening in order to formulate a screening schedule that takes into account your personal risk, your personal concerns, and your current state of health.

For example, the medical community has not reached a consensus on screening schedules for prostate cancer or for breast cancer. The American Cancer Society recommends that a man should begin discussing a personal schedule for prostate cancer screening with his physician starting at age 45 if he is African American or if he has a family history of prostate cancer. Otherwise, he should begin this discussion age 50. The Centers for Disease Control and Prevention and the National Cancer Institute also recommend that men discuss their personal risk factors and current state of health with their physician.

The American Cancer Society and the Centers for Disease Control and Prevention both recommend that women begin regular mammographic screening at age 40, while the National Cancer Institute defers regular screening to age 50

In both of these cases, and as a matter of fact for any cancer, your personal risk, family history, and current state of health are key factors to deciding the optimal screening schedule for you as an individual. In order to keep up to date with the latest recommendations, you should check the American Cancer Society Web site, the National Cancer Institute Web site, and the Centers for Disease Control and Prevention Web site for current recommendations. These Web sites are listed at the end of this chapter. You should discuss any of your personal concerns about developing cancer along with your family and personal history of cancer with your physician so that your personal screening schedule is optimized for you.

The American Cancer Society recommends periodic physical examinations by a doctor for cancer of the thyroid, oral cavity, skin, lymph nodes, testes, and ovaries in anyone over the age of 20.

Why is there disagreement about prostate cancer and breast cancer?

A specific screening schedule for prostate cancer is not recommended by the Centers for Disease Control and Prevention, the National Cancer Institute, or the American Cancer Society because the standard screening exam yields many false positives, which lead to unnecessary worry. It is also not clear whether treating men for low-grade low-stage prostate cancer benefits their lives relative to the side-effects that the treatment causes. This is especially true when these men have less than 10 years life expectancy because of other health problems.

Similarly, a recent study has shown that some women who undergo mammographic screening beginning at age 40 will undergo biopsies for false positive findings. In comparison, the study concluded that not enough lives were saved to account for the procedures performed. This study recommended that regular mammographic screening start at age 50 instead of age 40.

It is important to realize that these studies look at reduction of risk for the population as a whole and not for the individual. If you have a personal history of risk factors for breast cancer, if you have a family history of breast cancer, or if you have a personal concern about having breast cancer then you should discuss these factors with your physician. You could be a woman who will benefit from earlier screening.

Why isn't there a screening test for lung cancer or other cancers that are very aggressive?

Although lung cancer causes the most deaths from cancer today, a good screening test for lung cancer is not available now. Lung cancer has to be at least about 1 cm in size before it is detected on a chest x-ray. There are encouraging results from screening with spiral CT scans, according to a recent clinical trial. The problem is that many of the abnormalities that are discovered with these scans turn out not to be cancer on a biopsy. This means patients endure many unnecessary biopsies of the lung. Any recommendations that result from these clinical trials for screening methods will be based on statistics derived from many patients that prove that the screening method improves outcomes for patients with lung cancer.

Ovarian cancer is not a common cancer but it is the third-largest cause of cancer deaths in women. It is not easy to pick up at an early stage by physical examination, and most patients are diagnosed after it has metastasized to distant sites. There is active research to develop a screening test for ovarian cancer, and some tests have been developed that are geared to women who have a strong family history of ovarian cancer.

Are there experimental screening tests that I can try?

Cancer researchers are actively investigating now and improved screening tests. The National Cancer Institute has information on clinical trials that are specifically for cancer screening and that are supported by government funding. There are also Web sites that list clinical trials in general. In 2009 a new nonprofit Web site called ResearchMatch.org was introduced that tries to match people with clinical trials that meet their needs. These are all listed at the end of this chapter.

If you sign up for a clinical trial, be sure to ask how the test will be paid for. Insurance may not cover a clinical trial. Sometimes, but not always, the group sponsoring the trial will pay for it.

How often should I be screened?

The American Cancer Society, the Centers for Disease Control and Prevention, and the National Cancer Institute recommend schedules for cancer screening. Sometimes doctors prefer to perform screening more frequently, especially if there is a low side-effect profile. For example, there has been some suggestion that if you don't have one of the human papilloma viruses (HPV) viruses that is associated with cervical cancer, then you can wait every 2-3 years to get a Pap smear instead of annually. Statistics suggest that this is valid for many people, but there are deficits in this argument. For example, not all cervical cancers in older women are associated with HPV. A Pap smear may not be a full sweep of the cervix, and an abnormal area might be missed. In addition, the pathologist reading the Pap smear may not notice a subtle abnormality, which subsequently could give a cancer more time to spread.

Remember that your personal risk, family history, and current state of health are key factors to deciding the optimal screening schedule for you as an individual. You should discuss these factors with your physician so that your personal screening schedule is optimized for you. Be sure to check and see what your insurance will cover.

What is the rationale for screening tests and how often I should have one?

Screening recommendations are developed based on how likely the test is to detect someone with cancer. So, if breast cancer is unusual in women in their twenties, and mammograms pick up only 75 per cent of breast cancers, then mammograms will pick up only a very small number of women in their twenties. This is weighed against the risk of developing cancer from the increased radiation associated with the mammogram, the cost to the health system of performing so many negative mammograms (meaning no findings suspicious for cancer), and the cost of performing biopsies on false positive findings (meaning findings suspicious for cancer that turn out to not be cancer).

If no one in my family has had breast or colon cancer, should I undergo the recommended screening tests?

As was mentioned in the previous chapter, most cases of breast and colon cancer are not familial and so most patients who develop cancer will not have a family history of cancer. That means that it is important for everyone to undergo screening tests once he or she reaches the recommended starting age. I have been asked the question, "If no one in my family has ever had colon cancer, should I undergo screening according to the recommended schedule, which means a colonoscopy at age 50?" The answer is *Yes*. If you do have a strong family history, you might need to start screening before you are 50 years old. The same is true for breast cancer. If you have a strong family history you may need to start having mammograms before age 35, even if you have not been diagnosed as having a gene such as BRCA1 or BRCA2, either of which is known to elevate your risk. By strong I mean that several first-degree relatives have been diagnosed with the same cancer. A first-degree relative is a parent, a sibling, or a child. So if your mother and your older sister were diagnosed with breast cancer, you should discuss this with your physician and you may want to adjust the schedule of your screening mammograms.

At what age should I stop having screening tests?

The answer to this question depends upon how healthy you are, how much longer you could be expected to live, and how aggressive the cancer type you are screening for could be. Prostate cancer is often a slow-growing cancer, especially in elderly men with no family history. If you do not think you will live for another 10 years because you have another serious health condition, then you may not want to be screened for prostate cancer. This is especially the case if you are either not healthy enough or simply not willing to undergo therapy. You should consult with your physician before making a final decision.

25

The other thing to take into consideration is that even if you might not live for many more years, what would be the downside of not getting a screening test? Even if you would not want aggressive therapy, you might consider a limited form of treatment to prevent a high-grade cancer from spreading and affecting your quality of life. For example, breast cancer often metastasizes to the bone, which can be very painful and debilitating. If a breast cancer is small and localized, it can be easily surgically removed and reduce any chance of spreading to distant sites. You might make the choice not to undergo chemotherapy, but you could benefit from the removal of the main, primary tumor.

Does a positive screening test mean I have cancer?

It depends upon the screening test. Only screening tests that include a biopsy can give you an actual diagnosis of cancer. Of the screening tests currently recommended by the American Cancer Society, only cervical screening, colonoscopy and uterine cancer screening include a biopsy. If the biopsy is read as cancer and it is accurate, then you do have cancer. A biopsy might show atypia, dysplasia, or *in situ* cancer. In that case, a repeat-biopsy, more frequent surveillance, or a treatment to ablate the abnormality might be recommended.

Mammography and the PSA blood test for breast and prostate cancer, respectively, are indirect tests for cancer, and therefore alone they cannot render a diagnosis of cancer. If a mammogram or PSA-level screening test is called positive, then you have an increased likelihood of having cancer, but you do not have cancer until a biopsy proves it.

What do I do if I have a positive PSA-level screening test for prostate cancer?

Your blood PSA levels can be elevated after exercise, if you have benign hypertrophy of the prostate (BPH, a very frequent condition as men get older), or if you have an infection of the prostate. Putting the results together with your risk factors, such as whether or not you have had cancer in this site before, how old you are, your family's cancer history, etc., then your physician will recommend either that you have a biopsy or that you have a repeat screening test in the near future. Prostate cancer is usually slow-growing; therefore, if the likelihood factor from the screening test is low or intermediate, and you have no family history of prostate cancer, then repeat screening might be the best recommendation.

What do I do if I have a positive mammogram?

There is a rating system for the abnormalities in mammograms that measures how likely the abnormality is to be cancer. It is called the BIRADS number, and ranges from 1 to 5. (The acronym *BIRADS* stands for Breast Imaging Reporting and Data System.) Women with a BIRADS of 4 or 5 are recommended to have a biopsy. Women with a BIRADS of 1 or 2 are not, unless there are other reasons to suspect the abnormality is breast cancer. Women with a BIRADS of 3 are in the gray zone. If you have a BIRADS of 3, your doctors should consider your personal risk factors, such as whether or not you have had cancer in this site before, how old you are, your family's cancer history, etc., and then recommend either that you have more tests, that you possibly undergo a biopsy, or that you have a repeat screening test in the near future, usually within 3 to 6 months.

Does a negative screening test mean I do not have cancer?

It depends on the test. Screening tests are rated on how *sensitive* or *specific* they are. A *sensitive* test is one that tries to minimize false negatives in order to minimize the number of patients who really do have cancer but who are not caught by the test—that is, who have a negative screening test result. A *specific* test is one that tries to minimize false positives, so that the follow-up biopsies that

27

are not going to have cancer in them, and therefore are not necessary, are minimized. Sometimes it is hard to find a test that is both *highly sensitive* and *highly specific*. In general, specificity is sacrificed in favor of sensitivity in the United States. This results in more false positives and unnecessary biopsies but also results in fewer patients whose cancers are missed.

Can the symptoms of cancer help it to be detected early?

This depends upon the type of cancer. Uterine cancer usually causes unexpected vaginal bleeding. This symptom, especially in a post-menopausal woman, should be treated like a positive screening test and means that she should see a doctor for further testing, including possibly a biopsy. Blood in the urine can also be caused by cancer, but it is not a particularly specific symptom. Lumps or masses in the breast that are discovered by self-examination should be reported to your doctor for follow-up testing. Also, visual changes in color, size, and shape of moles are possible signs of melanoma, a form of cancer. These should also be examined by a doctor, in this case a dermatologist.

What should I do if my doctor thinks that I need another test based on a positive screening result?

If you have a symptom that has put you in a category in which you may have an increased likelihood of having cancer, you will need to make a decision about further testing. One option is to go forward with the next step. You may also want to consider a second opinion. Never, ever shy away from getting a second opinion; they are common practice. You can get a second opinion and bring the resulting recommendations to your local doctor so that you can continue your testing close to home.

Some cancers are known to be very aggressive, and others are known to be very labile (meaning slow to get bigger or spread), and others are in-between. When interpreting screening results, some doctors are very conservative, meaning they want a more definitive test, especially if the cancer type under consideration is aggressive. The most definitive test is a tissue biopsy, which is discussed in the next chapter (**Chapter 4. How is cancer diagnosed?**) Other patients are more comfortable with a wait and see approach, especially if the cancer type under consideration is very labile (slow to grow larger in size or to spread).

In the United States, approximately 80 per cent of breast biopsies based on mammographic screening are negative. In England, this ratio is almost reversed. Women in England are reported as being angry if they are put through the process of getting a biopsy and it is negative. This difference results from the bias toward a more *sensitive* result in the United States compared to a bias toward a more *specific* result in England when considering the cut-off in the BIRADS number to use for recommending a biopsy. You have to decide for yourself if having a negative result would upset you or would make you feel relieved. Important to making this decision are the last two questions—what is the downside if I don't have this test now, and what is the downside if I do.

Where can I get a second opinion?

You can get a second opinion from a cancer hospital. There are institutions called cancer centers across the United States that specialize in cancer research and treatment. Cancer centers can apply to the National Cancer Institute (NCI) for designation as an NCI Cancer Center, or the even higher-level designation of NCI Comprehensive Cancer Center, depending on how much research they do and how many clinical trials they carry out. A list of cancer centers and their location is maintained by the NCI on their Web site. The magazine *US News and World Report* reviews cancer hospitals and ranks them according to their excellence. These Web sites and others with information about hospitals and centers that specialize in cancer are listed at the end of this chapter. This information can help you.

Now, what if you are in a remote area far from a cancer center? I would recommend finding the closest large medical center that you can easily travel to, and selecting someone there to see. It is useful to see a doctor who has more experience in the field, or who works in a practice of multiple doctors where they talk informally among themselves, or even hold weekly conferences, in order to reach a consensus on how to approach the gray-area cases.

As mentioned above, you can get a second opinion and bring the recommendations to your local doctor so that you can continue your testing close to home.

Is it OK not to want to get a screening test if I am healthy and in the recommended age range for screening?

What I would like to talk about here is denial, or sometimes just procrastination. It is very easy to delay a screening test because you're just too busy (procrastination) or because you'd rather not know when you suspect there might be a problem (denial). Remember, not everyone gets cancer but anyone *can* get cancer. It is important to put that screening test in an important place of your mind. You might put it off for months, but don't put it off for years.

You should also sit down and review your health insurance, your disability insurance, and your life insurance. You should be comfortable with your sense of preparedness for a diagnosis. If you are considering retiring, you must review your insurance options. If you have a strong family history you definitely need to keep your insurance in a prepared state. Even if you don't have a family history of cancer, you need to consider the possibility of developing cancer. Find an insurance policy that will cover the cost of treating cancer.

Web sites for information on screening recommendations

http://cancer.org Maintained by the American Cancer Society. Go to this Web site and search for screening or early detection.

http://cdc.gov Maintained by the Centers for Disease Control and Prevention. Go to this Web site and search for preventive cancer screening.

http://www.cancer.gov Maintained by the National Cancer Institute. Go to this Web site, scroll down to Cancer Topics, and click on the link to *Screening And Testing.*

Web sites for current research and clinical trials to screen for a specific type of cancer

http://www.cancer.gov Maintained by the National Cancer Institute with listings by cancer type. For example, for lung cancer screening trials go to http://www.cancer.gov , scroll down to Cancer Topics, click on the link to *Screening And Tests*, and then click on the link to *Lung Cancer: Screening And Testing.* Scroll down and look for a link to clinical trials for screening tests under study.

Web sites for information on clinical trials in general

http://EmergingMed.com Maintained by an Internet information company that receives subscription fees from pharmaceutical and biotechnology companies to publish their trial information.

http://ClinicalTrials.gov Maintained by the National Library of Medicine, a sister institute to the National Cancer Institute. Both are institutes within the National Institute of Health.

Web sites for information on clinical trials in general, continued

http://www.cancer.gov/clinicaltrials/search/   A search engine for trial information maintained by the National Cancer Institute

http://ResearchMatch.org A nonprofit Web site designed to match up patients with ongoing clinical trials. ResearchMatch is a Clinical and Translational Science Award initiative funded by the National Center for Research Resources, a sister institute to the National Cancer Institute. Both are institutes within the National Institute of Health.

http://CenterWatch.com Maintained by an Internet information company that receives subscription fees from pharmaceutical and biotechnology companies to publish their trial information.

http://SearchClinicalTrials.org Maintained by a nonprofit organization called Center for Information and Study on Clinical Research Participation.

http://www.cancertrialshelp.org/   Maintained by the National Cancer Institute Clinical Trials Cooperative Groups.

http://cancer.org maintained by the American Cancer Society. Search for clinical trials.

http://www.nccn.org/clinical_trials/patients.asp Maintained by the National Cancer Center Network of cancer centers that are designated by the National Cancer Institute, and many of which are comprehensive cancer centers.

http://www.marycrowley.org A research foundation whose goal it is to make personalized therapy an option for every patient. They offer clinical trials that are focused on targeted therapies.

Web sites for information on clinical trials in general, continued
http://trp.cancer.gov/ A list of institutions that have a Specialized Program of Research Excellence (SPORE) grant awarded by the National Cancer Institute and focused on a specific type of cancer. These research groups often have clinical trials in progress.

Web sites to find a place to seek a second opinion
http://www.cancer.gov/researchandfunding/extramural/can cercenters Maintained by the National Cancer Institute (NCI) and has information defining the cancer centers and a tool to find a cancer center near you. A list of NCI designated cancer centers and comprehensive cancer centers and their location can be found at this site http://www.cancer.gov/researchandfunding/extramural/can cercenters/find-a-cancer-center .

http://health.usnews.com/sections/health/ Maintained by the magazine *US News and World Report.* This site reviews cancer centers and ranks them according to their excellence (go to the Web site and either search for a link to the Best Hospital for Cancer or locate the link on the page for Best Hospital by Specialty and choose Cancer.

http://www.nccn.org/ Maintained by the National Cancer Center Network of cancer centers. The NCCN member cancer centers are listed under Patient Resources, or use the site search engine to search for Member Cancer Centers.

http://www.marycrowley.org A research foundation whose goal it is to make personalized therapy an option for every patient. They offer clinical trials that are focused on targeted therapies.

Web sites to find a place to seek a second opinion, continued

http://trp.cancer.gov/ A list of institutions that have a Specialized Program of Research Excellence (SPORE) grant awarded by the National Cancer Institute and focused on a specific type of cancer. Institutions with a SPORE award in, for example, breast cancer will have a large community of specialists dealing with breast cancer.

http://www.aaci-cancer.org/ The official Web site for the American Association of Cancer Centers and whose mission is to promote the common interests of cancer centers. It maintains a membership directory. Cancer Centers can become members whether they have NCI designation or not.

Information to discuss with your doctor if you are not sure how often you should be screened for a type of cancer.

Personal Risk of Cancer will include exposure history, for example, cigarette smoking history, occupational history, and any previous diagnosis of abnormality in a screening test, such as abnormal cells on a Pap smear.

Family History will include a detailed family tree in which you note anyone who died of cancer and at what age, to the best of your knowledge. Relatives related by blood are important; in-laws do not count.

Your current state of health.

Information to discuss with your doctor if you are not sure how often you should be screened for a type of cancer, continued.

Your concerns about developing cancer and about being tested or treated for cancer.

Questions for your doctor if you have a positive screening test.

What are all the risk factors that suggest a diagnosis of cancer, and what are the ones that don't?

Questions for your doctor if you have a positive screening test, continued.

How accurate is this screening test, or this symptom that I have, in predicting that I have cancer?

What will happen in the next test—can it harm me at all?

How accurate is the next test?

What will happen if I want to wait and see—is this usually a slow-growing, less aggressive type of tumor, or should I act fast on this information?

What will happen next if I want to proceed and get the next test?

Chapter 4. How is cancer diagnosed?

Terms discussed in this chapter (listed alphabetically)
Biopsy
Clinical stage
Core needle biopsy
Excisional biopsy
Exploratory surgery
Fine needle aspiration
First-time diagnosis
Incisional biopsy
Laparoscopic surgery
NCI cancer centers
Pathologic stage
Primary tumor
Recurrence
SPORE awards
TNM stage

Is this a first-time diagnosis of a cancer or a recurrence?

First, it helps to know how your doctor determined that you have cancer, and what evidence he or she has for it. The first time someone tells you that you have a certain type of cancer, it should be a diagnosis based on an evaluation showing there are malignant cells, either in solid tissue sections or in fluid.

This is different from diagnosing a recurrence, which might be determined by measuring the quantity of a protein that your cancer cells excrete. For example, if you have ovarian cancer, and your ovarian cancer releases a protein called Cancer Antigen 125 (CA-125), then your blood level of CA-125 should diminish after surgery. At this point, your doctor may use the CA-125 level in your blood as an indirect measurement of whether your cancer has returned.

But, the first time you are diagnosed with a cancer, it should be because a pathologist has seen cancer cells in some tissue or body fluid that has been taken for diagnostic purposes. This is referred to as a *tissue diagnosis*.

Sometimes people develop more than one type of cancer. In this case, there should be a first-time diagnosis for the second cancer. It is not a recurrence and it will also need a tissue diagnosis. If you have had breast cancer and your doctor is concerned that you have kidney cancer, then he or she will need a tissue diagnosis to demonstrate that it is kidney cancer. If you have had breast cancer in one breast, and a new cancer appears in the other breast, it could be either a recurrence or a new incidence of breast cancer in the other breast. In that case a biopsy is usually performed and compared to the previous breast cancer to see if the second one is a new incidence, referred to as a new *primary*, or a recurrence.

How is a first-time diagnosis of cancer made?

A first-time diagnosis is made by examining cells or a fragment of tissue from the abnormal area. The cells are usually obtained from a biopsy. There are three different types of biopsies: fine needle aspiration, core biopsy, and surgical biopsy. Cells for examination might also be obtained from fluid removed from the patient, such as a blood sample, a urine sample, a spinal fluid sample, fluid around the lungs or the heart, or fluid in the abdomen. Any cells present are filtered from the fluid and examined.

If a biopsy cannot be performed without major surgery, then the patient will undergo exploratory surgery and the surgeon will take out a piece of the abnormal area. Often the surgeon will ask the pathologist to look at a *frozen section* for a preliminary diagnosis or to make sure that there is enough tissue in the biopsy to make a diagnosis. This is a sample of tissue that bypasses the more complicated processing that tissue goes through before it can be put onto a slide for examination under the

37

microscope. It means that a small section of the biopsy can be examined within about 20 minutes of being removed from the patient.

Sometimes surgery will start out as exploratory, and will switch to a surgery to remove as much tumor as possible. In this case, the patient is asked in advance to consent to undergo a larger, definitive surgery to try to take out all of the tumor if the frozen section is cancer.

In the past, major exploratory surgery was the standard method for diagnosing many types of cancer. However, in recent years computed tomographic (CT)-guided fine needle aspiration and laparoscopy have been introduced as a means of getting tissue from deep areas to evaluate patients for cancer. For example, exploratory surgery of the abdomen used to be the mainstay for diagnosing ovarian cancer. However, many centers now perform laparoscopy if they think that the tumor has not spread far into the abdomen. As a patient, you should explore the various means of getting tissue for diagnosis that are being suggested to you. It is also important to work with a surgeon and a center that are experienced in performing laparoscopies in order to make sure tumor is accidentally seeded into area that it had not yet spread to.

What is a fine needle aspiration biopsy?

Biopsies can come from many different procedure types that produce different amounts of material for a pathologist to look at, and therefore have varying accuracy. A small needle, about the size of the needle used for a flu vaccine, can be injected, and loosened cells are removed for diagnosis. This is called a fine needle aspiration. Fine needle aspirations, commonly referred to as FNA, are very small, but many times they are adequate for diagnosis and give sufficient information to plan the appropriate next step in staging and treatment.

What is a core biopsy?

A larger needle can remove a sliver of tissue called a core, which shows different types of cells and the manner in which they congregate and interact. Core biopsies are typically guided by radiological imaging, and these can be very effective in providing a diagnosis so that the next step in staging and treatment can be planned.

What is a surgical biopsy?

Larger surgical biopsies might be performed to get more tissue for diagnosis. This will be either an incisional or an excisional biopsy. An *incisional* biopsy is one where an incision is made into the tumor and some of the suspicious mass is removed. Brain tumors are a special case in which incisional biopsies are performed to take out a little bit of the lesion to see what it is.

An *excisional* biopsy attempts to remove the entire tumor and some normal tissue around it so that as the piece of tumor is pulled out of the body, it cannot leave behind any tumor cells along its tract that might seed a new tumor.

What kind of biopsy should I have?

It depends on the organ system. For the most common cancers, the following types of biopsies are recommended. For lung cancer, a bronchoscopy with a small incisional biopsy; or a CT-guided FNA or CT-guided core biopsy is preferred. The choice depends upon whether the suspicious mass is in an airway that can be reached by bronchoscopy or not.

For breast cancer, a fine needle aspiration or a core biopsy is preferred over an excisional biopsy. When excisional biopsies are performed, the surgeon is trying to take out as little tissue as possible, not knowing if the patient has cancer, and frequently they do not get out all of the cancer. This means that the patient has to undergo a second surgery. The American College of Surgeons recommends against an excisional biopsy as a first-line biopsy for breast cancer.

An FNA is appropriate if the tumor is large and there is no question that it might be *in situ*. FNAs cannot differentiate *in situ* from invasive cancer. FNAs are used to biopsy lymph nodes to determine the stage of the cancer if there are large lymph nodes that are very suspicious. The size of the lymph nodes are evaluated by ultrasounding the tissue of the armpit.

For colon cancer the standard is a colonoscopy with biopsy of any polyps. This is usually straightforward and gives enough information. For prostate cancer, several core biopsies performed on the right and left lobes are the standard of care. There is no incisional or excisional biopsy done here.

What information do you get from a biopsy?

The pathologist will determine which category the cells belong in—are they normal, atypical, dysplastic, *in situ*, borderline, or invasive/malignant cancer? Anything dysplastic, *in situ*, borderline, or invasive is typically given a grade as described in Chapter 1. If there is invasive cancer, then the pathologist will also determine whether this is a primary cancer, i.e. whether it is native to the organ that has been biopsied, or whether it comes from a distant part of the body and has metastasized to this organ.

For example, if you have fluid around your heart with cancer cells in it, then they most likely came from someplace other than your heart. The cells can be tested to see if they are heart muscle cells or not. If they are not heart muscle cells, you will undergo further testing to identify the primary cancer that has metastasized to the pericardial space, the space that lines the heart.

A mass in the liver may be either a primary liver cancer or a metastasis. This is determined by the radiographic imaging studies of the liver, by the characteristics of the cells under the microscope, and by special tests that can be performed on the cells and interpreted by the pathologist. If you have a biopsy from the colon and it looks like colon cancer, then this is typically considered to be a colonic primary. The presence of dysplastic cells in the lining of the colon supports the diagnosis of a primary colonic tumor (dysplasia was described in Chapter 1)

How do the doctors decide what my stage is, that is how far my tumor has spread?

The next important piece of information is determining how far the tumor has spread. As noted in Chapter 1, stage is not important in brain cancer, in leukemia, or in lymphoma. Prognostic information for leukemias and lymphomas relies most heavily on the type of tumor and, in some cases, the grade. For brain cancer the most important prognostic factor is the type of cancer (based on its cell type), its grade, and the location of the tumor.

But stage is an important prognostic factor for almost every other cancer type. The extent of spread can be quantified using the staging system developed by the American Joint Commission on Cancer (AJCC). This staging system is based on T, the tumor size or how many layers it has invaded through, N, which is based on the involvement of regional lymph nodes, and M, which is based simply on whether or not there have been distant metastases. (See the section titled **Are all metastases equal as a sign of aggressiveness?** in **Chapter 1. What is cancer?** for a definition of regional lymph node metastases versus distant metastases.) The T stage is typically an integer ranging from 1 to 4, N is an integer ranging from 0 to 3, and M is either 0 (no distant metastases) or 1 (there are distant metastases).

For every tumor that has a TNM staging system, there is an algorithm for determining an overall stage based on the individual TNM values. Overall stage is expressed in Roman numerals I to IV where I has the best prognosis for the AJCC stage algorithms. Any tumor with an M value of 1 is a stage IV tumor.

Other staging systems exist, such as the Dukes-Collier staging method for colon cancer. This is expressed as

41

capital letters A to D where A has the best prognosis. I will use the AJCC type of stages to describe how decisions are made. (Note that there is a one-to-one correspondence between AJCC and other staging systems for most cancers. For example a Duke's Stage D colon cancer is an AJCC Stage IV colon cancer.)

What is the difference between pathological stage and clinical stage?

Before surgery, the *clinical stage* is estimated from radiology studies based on the estimated size of the tumor (clinical T stage); whether enlarged lymph nodes can be seen (clinical N stage); and whether there are abnormalities elsewhere (clinical M stage). The M status can come from imaging, e.g. MRI or CT-scan. A clinical AJCC stage can be estimated from these measurements and observations.

After surgery, the pathologist measures the exact size of the tumor for the T stage in the tissue removed from the patient (pathologic T stage) and ascertains the number of nodes involved for the N stage (pathologic N stage). This direct measurement of T and N are the basis for the pathologic AJCC stage in cases in which there is no evidence of distant metastases, i.e. M is 0. If M is 1 based on imaging, then the patient will have a clinical Stage IV tumor. A pathologic stage measurement is more accurate than a clinical stage, especially for low-stage tumors.

Should I opt only for pathological stage before I am treated?

No. Currently, treatment plans more often include chemotherapy or radiation therapy before surgical resection. Since the tumor will shrink in size with this treatment, the initial assessment of stage will be mostly clinical. Patients receive such therapy before surgery for two reasons. One is to shrink the tumor so that the surgery will be easier. The second is to see how the patient's cancer is responding to the type of therapy that is being given. If there is not a complete disappearance of the cancer, then the type of therapy might be changed after the surgery so that tumor cells resistant to the therapy given before surgery are treated. This approach is known as giving *neo-adjuvant* therapy to the patient. Treatments given after surgery are called *adjuvant* therapy.

Should I consider a second opinion for my diagnosis?

Second opinions are very important for an interesting reason. It has been estimated that there is a major change in approximately 10 to 15 per cent of material sent for a second opinion. For instance, some inflammatory conditions can mimic cancer. Lung biopsies can have abnormal-looking cells that are "beaten-up" by pneumonia and look like cancer cells. And reassessments with a second opinion can have important practical implications. Just recently, a man who thought he had only a few months to live found out 2 years later that he had chronic pancreatitis, not pancreatic cancer. This was great news for him, but he learned it after he had quit his job and spent his entire savings on living it up. *That* part was not great.

Where can I get a second opinion?

You can use the same resources that were given for a second opinion on your screening test to ask for a second opinion on your diagnostic material. These are found under useful Web sites for seeking a second opinion that are listed at the end of this chapter. You can also ask your doctor to ask the pathologists who interpreted your diagnosis to send the material to the expert that they use for consultation on difficult cases. Remember—seeking a second opinion does not mean you have to transfer all your care to a distant hospital if you want to be treated close to home. You can have the second opinion and any recommendations sent to your local doctor.

Another way to get information about where to send pathology material for a second opinion is to search for institutions that have a Specialized Program of Research

43

Excellence (SPORE) grant focused on the type of cancer that you have been diagnosed with—for example a SPORE grant award in breast cancer. These grants are awarded by the NCI to institutions to support the advancement of basic research into new clinical trials. In order to receive an award, the institution must demonstrate in its application that it serves a large patient population for that cancer type and that it has experts in pathology, surgery, radiology, and both medical and radiation oncology in that field. The SPORE awards also support a patient advocate program at each site and can be a source of patient-support and advocacy groups.

An important thing to remember when you get a diagnosis of cancer is that cancers range from something that is very easy to treat to cancers that are very aggressive. You can review the statistics on your cancer at the American Cancer Society Web site and at the Surveillance Epidemiology and End Results Web site maintained by the NCI (see list of useful Web sites for statistics at the end of this chapter.

What if I get a second opinion and the second pathologist does not agree with the first pathologist about the tumor diagnosis? Or about the grade? Or about whether it is malignant or not?

Differences in grade are important, and these are not uncommon. My advice would be to take the grade assigned by the pathologist(s) who see this type of tumor more or most often. A difference in opinion as to whether a tumor is non-malignant or malignant is critical to your treatment plan, and to your sense of well-being. Consider obtaining an opinion from the pathologist(s) who see these cases most often. You can ask for a third opinion. Again, your doctor can recommend someone, or your pathology department can recommend someone, or you can try the top 10 cancer centers or a cancer center with a SPORE grant award for that cancer type.

Web sites for cancer statistics to learn how aggressive, or how indolent, your cancer is

http://seer.cancer.gov/ The Surveillance Epidemiology and End Results (SEER) published by the National Cancer Institute.

http://seer.cancer.gov/statistics/ Statistics in the Surveillance Epidemiology and End Results (SEER) published by the National Cancer Institute. Select the link to SEER Cancer Statistics Review for the years most recently reviewed and published (under the headline Annual reports and Monographs).

http://cancer.org Maintained by the American Cancer Society.

Web sites to find a place to seek a second opinion

http://www.cancer.gov/researchandfunding/extramural/cancercenters Maintained by the National Cancer Institute (NCI) and has information defining the cancer centers and a tool to find a cancer center near you. A list of NCI designated cancer centers and comprehensive cancer centers and their location can be found at this site http://www.cancer.gov/researchandfunding/extramural/cancercenters/find-a-cancer-center .

http://health.usnews.com/sections/health/ Maintained by the magazine *US News and World Report*. This site reviews cancer centers and ranks them according to their excellence (go to the Web site and either search for a link to the Best Hospital for Cancer or locate the link on the page for Best Hospital by Specialty and choose Cancer.

http://www.nccn.org/ Maintained by the National Cancer Center Network of cancer centers. The NCCN member cancer centers are listed under Patient Resources, or use the site search engine to search for Member Cancer Centers.

http://trp.cancer.gov/ A list of institutions that have a Specialized Program of Research Excellence (SPORE) grant awarded by the National Cancer Institute and focused on a specific type of cancer. Institutions with a SPORE award in, for example, breast cancer will have a large community of specialists dealing with breast cancer.

http://www.aaci-cancer.org/ The official Web site for the American Association of Cancer Centers and whose mission is to promote the common interests of cancer centers. It maintains a membership directory. Cancer Centers can become members whether they have NCI designation or not.

Questions to ask before a biopsy

What kind of biopsy will this be: fine needle aspiration, core biopsy, or incisional or excisional biopsy?

Which kind of biopsy does the American College of Surgeons recommend for the type of cancer that I might have?

Will you get enough information from the biopsy to plan surgery if I do have cancer?

Do they perform this type of biopsy regularly at this hospital or clinic?

Questions to ask after a biopsy

What is my diagnosis?

What organ did the cancer originate in?

What is the name of the type of cancer that I have?

Questions to ask after a biopsy, continued
Is it a special subtype?

How aggressive is this cancer type? What is the grade?

How far has this cancer spread? What is my stage? Is it a clinical stage (an estimate) or pathologic stage?

How accurate is my diagnosis?

Where can I send my slides for a second opinion?

Do I need surgery (or more surgery)?

Would I benefit from chemotherapy before surgery to remove the tumor?

Do I need treatment after surgery?

Reports you should ask your doctor for
Pathology reports
Radiology reports

Chapter 5. What is a sentinel lymph node biopsy?

> **Terms discussed in this chapter (listed alphabetically)**
> Isolated tumor cells in a lymph node
> Mediastinoscopy
> Sentinel lymph node biopsy

Patients who have been diagnosed with cancer get staged, as described in the previous chapter. To recap, the majority of tumors have a TNM stage based on tumor size (T), the extent of lymph node involvement (N), and the presence or absence of distant metastases (M). Lymph node status is important to assessing lung, colon, prostate, and breast cancer. It is also important in endometrial, ovarian, cervical, testicular, and skin cancer. It is *not* important for brain tumors.

What is lymph node status or the extent of lymph node involvement and why is it important?

We have an extensive drainage system in our body to drain excess fluid away from our tissues and special organs, and to return it to our blood vessels. I say return because fluid is constantly leaking from our blood vessels, and then it drains through the lymphatic system and gets returned into the bloodstream.

Lymph nodes are pieces of tissue about the size of a lentil or a small bean that are interspersed along what is called the lymphatic chain. Lymph nodes contain an orderly assembly of white blood cells that act like a sand filter for the fluid. Little bits of debris, bacteria, or tumor cells that are traveling in the lymphatic system get stuck in this filter. There are white blood cells that recognize something to be foreign to the system—a cell without a passport, so to speak. This might be a bacterial cell.

Sometimes our bodies are good at recognizing tumor cells as an abnormal population. The recognition cells will start a cascade of events designed to fight off the invader. If they are successful, then the tumor cell will be induced to undergo a process call *apoptosis,* which means that cell is triggered to commit suicide and die. So, if a vigilant lymph node picks up some tumor cells, it may be able to make them commit suicide. If not, then these cells might grow and divide, and create a metastasis.

Looking at lymph nodes is important for at least three reasons. First, lymph nodes let us know if the cancer cells are breaking away from the primary cancer and spreading to other parts of the body. Second, if there is a well-established metastasis in the lymph node as opposed to a few cells, then we know that this cancer is able to travel, to resist apoptosis, *and* to go on dividing in a foreign territory. The cancer cells thus have both a passport to travel and a visa to stay and live abroad. Finally, looking at the lymph nodes lets us know how much more cancer is in the patient, called the cancer burden. So we remove the lymph nodes to assess the ability of a cancer to metastasize and to reduce cancer burden.

Are there any side-effects to removing a chain of lymph nodes?

Removing a chain of lymph nodes disrupts the drainage system in that part of the body. If it has to be done to remove cancer, then so be it, it gets done. However, if you have a whole section of lymph nodes removed and there is no cancer in them, you did not benefit from cancer removal but you will have swelling problems in the area that that lymphatic chain used to drain for the rest of your life.

Is there a way to know that there is no cancer in the lymph nodes without having to remove a whole section of them?

The way that doctors have learned to avoid taking out a whole section of lymph nodes is to identify one or a few lymph nodes that are the first ones in the drainage route from the main cancer area. These are called *sentinel*

49

lymph nodes and they can be thought of as a sentinel guard who will give us early warning of any cancer in the lymph nodes. If these sentinel lymph nodes have no cancer in them, then there is no cancer beyond them (the sand filter of white blood cells is very effective). The sentinel lymph nodes are detected by injecting a little bit of blue dye and a radioactive tracer into the tumor, and then following the radioactivity signal until you know where the sentinel lymph nodes are. The blue dye helps to identify the node or nodes in the tissue.

What kind of cancers prompt using a sentinel lymph node biopsy to avoid taking out a whole section of lymph nodes?

Sentinel lymph node biopsy is routinely performed for breast cancer and for melanoma. Of the many advances in cancer therapy in the last decade, I think that sentinel lymph node biopsy is one of the most important in terms of quality of life. I advise people to ask their surgeons if sentinel lymph node biopsy is offered anywhere for the cancer type that they have.

If sentinel lymph node biopsy can be performed for your cancer, and it is not performed at your hospital, then ask your surgeon where you can get a sentinel lymph node biopsy with your surgery. Alternatively, seek out one of the cancer centers designated by the NCI, or listed as the best cancer hospitals by *US News and World Report* (see useful Web sites at the end of this chapter)

Besides breast cancer or melanoma, are sentinel lymph node biopsies used in any other cancer?

It is currently under investigation for several cancers with preliminary good results for cervical cancer, vulvar cancer, prostate cancer, and cancer of the mouth. Results on stomach cancer are very preliminary at the time this book was going to print. A lymph node close to the prostate can be identified without the blue dye and radioactive tracer, and it is essentially always biopsied to see if there is cancer. However, this is not always the true sentinel lymph node for this area, and there is research into using dye and tracer to identify the best node to sample.

There are difficulties in identifying the sentinel lymph node in lung cancer, penile cancers, bladder cancer, and colon and rectal cancers. In the case of colon and rectal cancers, it may not be that important to preserve the lymph node chain, because in surgery for colon cancer a section of the colon is routinely removed with the lymph nodes that it drains to. Lymph node sampling for lung cancer is discussed further in the next question, because it is very important.

The NCI has a Web site with information about sentinel lymph node biopsy (see useful Web sites at the end of this chapter).

What about the role of lymph nodes in lung cancer?

In the case of lung cancer, endometrial cancer, and ovarian cancer, the entire lymphatic drainage bed cannot be removed, and surgeons sample the local lymph nodes. For lung cancer, it is important to obtain as representative a sample as possible. Lung tissue has a high density of blood vessels and has an extensive lymphatic drainage system. This helps to efficiently oxygenate blood and remove fluid in the lungs so that we can oxygenate our bodies efficiently. It also means that tumors of the lung can easily access the bloodstream and lymphatics, which are the typical highways that tumor cells use to spread elsewhere, and hence metastasize. Lung cancers that are small and have not demonstrated any spread to another location do not fare as well as their counterparts in breast and colon cancer. This is likely due to the fact that there has been an *occult* metastasis, which is "*medispeak*" for having spread to another site that is not large enough to be detected.

Sampling of lymph nodes can be done during the surgery to remove the lung with cancer in it, or by performing a procedure before the open lung surgery called mediastinoscopy. It has been shown that a better sampling of the lymph nodes, and thus better staging, is performed with mediastinoscopy. If you have lung cancer, ask your surgeon if they will perform a mediastinoscopy. Seek out a surgeon that performs mediastinoscopy if your own surgeon does not. Again, local cancer centers and hospitals, NCI-designated cancer centers and comprehensive cancer centers, and information from the *US News and World Report* on cancer hospitals can help you find a surgeon who will perform mediastinoscopy (see list of Web sites to find hospitals that specialize in cancer treatment at the end of this chapter).

Web site with general information about sentinel lymph node biopsy

http://www.cancer.gov/cancertopics/factsheet/Therapy/sentinel-node-biopsy This Web site is created by the National Cancer Institute.

Web sites to find hospitals that specialize in cancer treatment

http://www.cancer.gov/researchandfunding/extramural/cancercenters Maintained by the National Cancer Institute (NCI) and has information defining the cancer centers and a tool to find a cancer center near you. A list of NCI designated cancer centers and comprehensive cancer centers and their location can be found at this site http://www.cancer.gov/researchandfunding/extramural/cancercenters/find-a-cancer-center .

http://health.usnews.com/sections/health/ Maintained by the magazine *US News and World Report*. This site reviews cancer centers and ranks them according to their excellence (go to the Web site and either search for a link to the Best Hospital for Cancer or locate the link on the page for Best Hospital by Specialty and choose Cancer.

Web sites to find hospitals that specialize in cancer treatment, continued

http://www.nccn.org/ Maintained by the National Cancer Center Network of cancer centers. The NCCN member cancer centers are listed under Patient Resources, or use the site search engine to search for Member Cancer Centers.

http://trp.cancer.gov/ A list of institutions that have a Specialized Program of Research Excellence (SPORE) grant awarded by the National Cancer Institute and focused on a specific type of cancer. Institutions with a SPORE award in, for example, breast cancer will have a large community of specialists dealing with breast cancer.

http://www.aaci-cancer.org/ The official Web site for the American Association of Cancer Centers and whose mission is to promote the common interests of cancer centers. It maintains a membership directory. Cancer Centers can become members whether they have NCI designation or not.

Important questions for your doctor

Is there a sentinel lymph node biopsy procedure for this type of cancer?

Do you perform it at your hospital?

How long have you been performing a sentinel lymph node biopsy?

How many have you done?

(In the case of lung cancer) Do you perform a mediastinoscopy?

Important questions for your doctor, continued
(If you have a lymph node metastasis) Do I have a well-established lymph node metastasis, a micrometastasis, or isolated tumor cells? (see section **Are all metastases equal as a sign of aggressiveness?** in **Chapter 1 What is cancer?** for a discussion of isolated tumor cells)

Chapter 6. What are borderline tumors?

Terms discussed in this chapter
Borderline tumors/tumors of unknown malignant potential

What is a borderline tumor or a tumor of unknown malignant potential?

There are several different states that a normal cell might go through before it becomes invasive and malignant. The most important ones are dysplasia and *in situ* cancer, which were described in Chapter 1. There is another type of tumor called either a *borderline tumor* or a *tumor of unknown malignant potential.* Unlike dysplasia and *in situ* cancer, both of which cannot metastasize, borderline tumors are recognizable as invasive tumors, but on detecting them we don't know whether or not they will behave like a malignant cancer. Put plainly, these are tumors in a gray zone. Examination of the tissue by pathologists cannot place certain tumors in a non-malignant versus a malignant category. They are "'tweeners."

What kinds of borderline tumors are there?

There are many different types of borderline tumors. The most common types of borderline tumors are low-grade tumors in the brain, a set of tumors called borderline tumors of the ovary, the low-grade mucinous tumor of the appendix, atypical carcinoid tumors, adrenocortical tumors, some lymphomas, monoclonal gammopathy of unknown clinical significance, smooth muscle tumors of unknown malignant potential, melanomas of unknown malignant potential, and gastrointestinal tumors of unknown malignant potential.

In some tumor types, pathologists can lean in one direction or another, that is, they can indicate that the tumor is *more* likely or *less* likely to be malignant. This "leaning" is based on how big they are, how atypical they are, and how fast they are dividing. In other types, there is no way to know which ones might end up as a metastasis later and which ones will not.

We are working to develop more detailed diagnostic tests so that we can better divide the borderline tumors into those that are more likely to be malignant and those that are less likely to be malignant, or even cleanly divide the non-malignant from the malignant ones.

What should I do if I am diagnosed with a borderline tumor?

This brings me back to how important it can be to get a second opinion. Borderline tumors are neither terribly common nor vanishingly rare, but somewhere in-between. This means that they will be seen less often in smaller or community hospitals and more often in large, cancer-specific hospitals. One of the most important things that you can do is get a second opinion from a pathologist who specializes in borderline tumors. Again, there are experts in these various fields. Your doctor may be able to ask the pathologist who diagnosed your material to recommend an expert. If you cannot identify a set of pathologists who specialize in your diagnosis, then try the pathologists at a cancer center that studies cancers in that organ system or at that site (see the end of this chapter for a list of Web sites that you can use to locate hospitals that specialize in cancer treatment).

How are borderline tumors treated?

Treatment decisions will vary according to the tumor type. In most cases, resection of the borderline tumor is important. It is appropriate to remove the tumor so that it cannot spread if it is inclined to behave like a malignant cancer. If it is not malignant, it may actually transform into something malignant so, much like an *in situ* cancer, it should be removed.

Other treatments might destroy the borderline tumor, such as radiation. This, and even some less aggressive chemotherapy regimen, might be recommended, especially if it is difficult to surgically remove the entire tumor. For example borderline brain tumors might be treated with radiation or chemotherapy to insure that they will not recur and possibly transform. Gastrointestinal stromal tumors of unknown malignant potential can often be treated with a drug that controls their growth. If you are trying to make a decision about how to be treated, you can also consider traveling to one of these institutions to get an opinion on how you should be treated. You can have the recommendations sent back to your doctor at home so that you can be treated close to your home and family.

Web sites to find hospitals that specialize in cancer treatment

http://www.cancer.gov/researchandfunding/extramural/can cercenters Maintained by the National Cancer Institute (NCI) and has information defining the cancer centers and a tool to find a cancer center near you. A list of NCI designated cancer centers and comprehensive cancer centers and their location can be found at this site http://www.cancer.gov/researchandfunding/extramural/can cercenters/find-a-cancer-center .

http://health.usnews.com/sections/health/ Maintained by the magazine US News and World Report. This site reviews cancer centers and ranks them according to their excellence (go to the Web site and either search for a link to the Best Hospital for Cancer or locate the link on the page for Best Hospital by Specialty and choose Cancer.

Web sites to find hospitals that specialize in cancer treatment, continued

http://www.nccn.org/ Maintained by the National Cancer Center Network of cancer centers. The NCCN member cancer centers are listed under Patient Resources, or use the site search engine to search for Member Cancer Centers.

http://trp.cancer.gov/ A list of institutions that have a Specialized Program of Research Excellence (SPORE) grant awarded by the National Cancer Institute and focused on a specific type of cancer. Institutions with a SPORE award in, for example, breast cancer will have a large community of specialists dealing with breast cancer.

http://www.aaci-cancer.org/ The official Web site for the American Association of Cancer Centers and whose mission is to promote the common interests of cancer centers. It maintains a membership directory. Cancer Centers can become members whether they have NCI designation or not.

Questions for your doctor about borderline tumors/tumors of unknown malignant potential

What are my treatment options?

Would I get other treatment options at a different hospital or center?

Where are centers that specialize in this diagnosis?

How effective is each treatment for my grade of tumor?

What can happen if my tumor isn't completely removed using a non-surgical treatment?

How complicated is the surgery?

58

Questions for your doctor about borderline tumors/tumors of unknown malignant potential, continued

What are the side-effects of surgical and of non-surgical treatment?

How well can you detect a change in my tumor from pre-malignant or borderline to frankly malignant?

How likely is it that my tumor could become or actually is malignant?

How fast could my tumor become frankly malignant?

Chapter 7. How is cancer treated?

Terms discussed in this chapter (listed alphabetically)
Advocacy groups
Aggressive therapy
Alternative therapies
Biological therapy
Chemotherapy
Chronic therapy
Immunotherapy
Living will
NCI cancer centers
Palliative therapy
Patient advocates
Personalized therapy
Quality of life
Radiation therapy
Side-effects
Smiling
SPORE awards
Surgery
Targeted therapy

One of the biggest decisions to make once you have a diagnosis of cancer is on what kind of treatment that you and your doctor think is best for you. You should think of you and your doctor as a team—your doctor is the coach and you are the player. I want to stress over and over how important it is for you to choose a doctor that "works for you." Older, younger, male, female, loquacious, blunt, terse—they come in all varieties. Just as you would want to find the right coach to bring out your best talents, you want to find the right doctor to work with you on your most important health questions. If you are unsure about your treatment plan, you can visit a cancer hospital that specializes in treating your cancer. If you want to stay close to home for your treatment, you can have the recommendations sent to your doctor who is close to home so the two of you can work on a plan that you are committed to.

What levels of treatment are there for cancer?

Level of care can be roughly divided into three categories—aggressive treatment, chronic treatment, and palliative treatment. Over time, you may end up receiving each of these levels of therapy. Care can be delivered as surgery, to remove as much tumor as possible; medical therapy, as chemotherapy, biological therapy, immunotherapy, or targeted therapy; and radiation therapy.

What kinds of treatment are there for cancer?

As stated in the previous paragraph, the three main categories of therapy are surgery, medical therapy, and radiation therapy.

Surgery can be performed for diagnosis, prognosis, or tumor removal/debulking, or all three at the same time. As described earlier in Chapter 4, prognosis comes from pathological assessment of the tissues that are removed from a patient. The main types of medical therapy today are chemotherapy, biological therapy, immunotherapy, and targeted therapy.

- Chemotherapies are chemical agents that are designed to kill cancer cells.

- Biological therapies are biological agents that help your own body fight a disease. They might be hormones that interfere with the cancer cells.

- Immunotherapies stimulate the immune cells in your body to fight cancer cells.

- Targeted therapies selectively seek out a molecule that your cancer cells have in them or on their surface.

These terms arose somewhat separately and there is some overlap, so that it can sometimes be confusing to decide whether you are having biological therapy or immunotherapy, or a therapy that falls into both categories.

Radiation therapies are high-energy rays or particles that are emitted by radioactive substances and are focused on the tumor cells. These can be delivered as an external beam, a special high-dose localized and focused beam (brachytherapy), proton therapy, or radiation seeds that are implanted in an organ and designed so that the radiation does not go far beyond the territory of the cancer.

Sometimes patients receive neo-adjuvant therapy, also described in Chapter 4 as therapy before surgery. The tumor is diagnosed on a small biopsy. The patient's stage is determined from a combination of imaging by radiologists and biopsies read by pathologists. The physicians can assess the response of the tumor to the chemotherapy. This is usually done by following the patient's radiology scans (CT scan, MRI, mammograms, etc.) to see if the tumor is shrinking. After a certain number of treatment cycles, the primary tumor area is removed and evaluated by a pathologist for any pockets of residual tumor cells that escaped treatment. If there are some left, then an alternative therapy can be selected to go after these resistant tumor cells.

Will I always be offered chemotherapy or radiation therapy after surgical removal of a cancer?

No. If a tumor is small enough, and it has not spread to local and regional tissues or demonstrated the ability to survive in "foreign" tissue, then no further therapy might be appropriate. If the tumor has metastasized to regional lymph nodes or beyond, then, depending on how healthy you are and how old you are, you can be offered more aggressive therapy.

What is personalized therapy or personalized medicine?

Chemotherapy and radiation are general treatments that are offered to patients. However, we know that even the same type of cancer varies from person to person. If we could identify the molecules or genes that make cancer behave a certain way, and tailor a therapy to that particular molecular or gene, then we could begin to treat tumors on a "personal" level. To do this, we would have to detect the molecules or genes that we can target with a treatment, then prescribe the targeted therapy to patients whose cancers test positive for that molecular or gene. Some examples of targeted therapy are antibodies that bind to specific molecules on a cancer cell, such as the Her2neu receptor that is found in some breast cancers. Others include the class of drugs known as tyrosine kinase inhibitors that stop the activity of enzymes that are over-active in some types of cancer cells. There are several targeted therapies available now and many more in clinical trials.

Hence, by knowing the molecular or genetic characteristics of a person's cancer, the therapy could be tailored to target that patient's cancer. While this is the goal for treating cancer, the mainstay of treatments is still radiation and general chemotherapy drugs. If you are interesting in investigating targeted therapies that are not offered as a standard treatment protocol, then you may want to investigate a clinical trial (see **Chapter 8 What are clinical trials?**).

What is aggressive therapy?

Aggressive therapy is just what it sounds like—pulling out the big guns to fight an aggressive disease. Typically, therapy is chemotherapy or radiation or both. Chemotherapy is usually a combination of several drugs given in "cycles." It might also mean more surgery, or one of the new "molecularly targeted" therapies that tries to neutralize tumor cells by attacking a specific molecule that they produce. Aiming for a molecular target is like aiming for a specific lethal target in your tumor cells. The reason for a battery of drugs is that your cancer is usually made up of several subgroups of cell types, each of which might be resistant to one of the drugs and exquisitely sensitive to another one. By giving the drugs in combination, the likelihood is higher of wiping out all of the subgroups without giving them enough time to evolve into a cell type that is resistant to all of the drugs that you will be given.

Aggressive therapy also carries with it the side-effect profiles for all of the drugs you are given. It is important to be aware of these. They should not necessarily stop you from receiving aggressive therapy, but you should be informed about how you will feel during the therapy, and what kind of effects might be permanent. You may want to know just how many patients experience any side-effect you are concerned about on a permanent basis. This you will want to weigh against how much of your lifetime you will be likely to get back. The answer to these questions might be very easy. The younger and the healthier that you are, the more aggressive therapy that you can usually tolerate with a trade-off of more years gained. Still, it is important to know that side-effect profile. For patients who are more mature, say in their late seventies and older, the aggressive therapies can be very harsh. These can reduce quality of life without giving back as many years if the patient already has other health problems. For this reason, these patients might receive less cycles of therapy, or different types of medication, or they might choose not to receive any or as much of the therapy.

What if I am offered aggressive therapy and I don't want it?

This is a difficult sort of decision. I stress again how important it is to find a coach who can guide you through this decision process. Also, second opinions, even third opinions, can help to consolidate a decision.

As an example, a healthy 85-year-old woman asked me once whether she should have chemotherapy for a 2.1 cm invasive carcinoma of the breast. The cancer was very low-grade, meaning that it was less likely to come back after surgery. Her sentinel lymph node was negative, so it appeared to not have spread anywhere. The size was just above the cut-off (at 2 cm) where therapy is recommended even if nodes are negative. Even though this cutoff is applied to categorize tumors as small, medium, large, and extra-large, the range of sizes is actually continuous so that a 2.1 cm tumor is barely a medium tumor and very close to a small tumor.

What are the chances that her tumor will come back in 5 years? What are the chances she will develop heart failure or lose feeling in her fingers and feet from chemotherapy? This could be very high, especially if she already has some heart disease. Depending on how healthy she is right now, how much longer will she be likely to live to suffer from a recurrence of this cancer? In 5 years she will be 90. If you think you will live well into your nineties, it would seem reasonable to have some chemotherapy. One of the places that breast tumors go to is the bone, and chemotherapy would be a way of preventing bone metastases that are painful and can be disabling. On the other hand, you may feel as though quality of life in your eighties is more important than longevity, or you do not expect that longevity, so you might not want chemotherapy. This is when you need to ask your doctor what your chances are of having your tumor come back in the remainder of your lifetime, ask our doctor what the side-effects are of your treatment plan, and decide how long you want to live and the level of quality of life you want.

What if you are in your fifties, though, and you are diagnosed with a breast cancer that is well into the medium size range, and one small but well-established metastasis in a lymph node? There is a reasonable chance that this tumor will come back in another site if you don't get chemotherapy. Is it a 100% chance—well, thank goodness no. But it is not something that you can ignore either, and you have a lot of life left to live. It is important to understand what the implications of the lymph node metastasis are here—it does mean the capability of surviving and growing in a foreign tissue, and that is a dangerous property. This is when a physician will recommend aggressive therapy.

What if I have a small tumor and I want more aggressive therapy than is recommended?

There should be some reason why you should benefit from this therapy before you should expose yourself to the side-effects that you can encounter. There are cases of small breast cancers less than 1.0 cm in size, with no lymph node involvement, but which are very high-grade. Sometimes, particularly if the woman is pre-menopausal, doctors will offer and these women will prefer to receive several cycles of chemotherapy in order to eradicate any tumor cells hiding out someplace. Given the high grade of the cancer and the young age of the patient, this is an option that can be followed. The bottom line is, is there any evidence to support a benefit for you from this treatment?

What if I have a very advanced cancer and I want very aggressive therapy?

There is no doubt that this can be a very difficult time. When a tumor is very advanced in a young adult, there can be several different options, and several doctors might each recommend a different approach. This can be confusing. Sometimes it is important to step back and see this as a choice rather than as a confusing array of options. If no one doctor can give you any evidence to indicate that one of the choices is truly better than the other one, then ask yourself which is the one that you feel best about taking? Part of being an effective team player is feeling good about what you are doing. An important thing to take into account is, it may not work as well or for as long as you want it to, and there will be side-effects. But, whatever happens, you know that you chose the path that you wanted to take.

Having said that, in some cases a tumor has progressed to a state such that experience has proven that certain options take away quality of life and don't give back time. This is often the case with lung cancer. Sometimes patients with lung cancer that has spread want to have the lung with the primary tumor taken out. However, the tumor may have spread far enough that they would be giving up a part of their lungs without getting time back. In a case like this, even if you wanted surgery, it would not be fair to operate on you; the end result might be that you have a lesser quality of life with no benefit.

Maybe the choice is brain surgery to remove a metastasis versus letting go. How much function might you lose with the brain surgery versus how much time you might get back is a very important question to ask. How likely is it that they can really get the entire tumor out? Where in the brain is the metastasis and what does that part of the brain control?

What should I look out for while receiving aggressive therapy?

During the course of aggressive therapy, there are several things that the patient and his or her caregiver need to watch out for. These can very from one type of therapy to another. You should always make sure that you have a current list of things to watch out for from your doctor. The following is a general list of some of the side-effects that some patients experience, but this is not meant to replace the list you get from your doctor. Also, some patients are able to tolerate treatment without much impact while others have more serious reactions. The degree of side-effects that a patient experiences is very personal.

Low immunity, or the inability to fight off infections; anemia, or not having enough red blood cells to carry oxygen around the body; low platelets, or not being able to repair little nicks in the sides of blood vessels; dehydration, or not having enough fluid for your heart and kidneys to operate; and malnutrition, or not getting enough good food to help the body to renew normal cells that are affected by the chemotherapy are just some of the side-effects that you could develop. Chemotherapy typically kills cells that are dividing rapidly. Our red blood cell and our white blood cells are affected by chemotherapy as our body is constantly renewing these. Megakaryocytes, big "manufacturing" cells that pinch off platelets, which work as "caulking" agents to repair little nicks in blood vessels, are diminished. The lining of our gut from our mouth through our stomach and intestines is affected. Our intestines normally replace their lining cells every six days, and so they are affected by any chemotherapy agent that attacks dividing cells. Patients often develop sores and bleeding. Some patients experience diarrhea; others develop skin rashes. Taste can be affected. Some people can develop jaundice and turn yellow.

Dehydration affects many body functions. When dehydrated, patients can become dizzy, overly sleepy, confused, and unable to walk properly. The electrolytes, or salts, in our bloodstream can get out of balance. The different salt concentrations play a vital role in charging up our cell batteries in our muscles, including and perhaps most importantly, the heart muscle.

For immunity, blood counts are important during therapy. Minor infections can become life-threatening while immunity is low. Signs of an infection should be reported to your doctor. For anemia and low platelets, our blood counts help monitor the affects of chemotherapy and radiation.

What are signs that anyone can recognize that show how affected a patient is from chemotherapy? Anemic patients become pale. This is best seen by looking at their conjunctiva, the lining between the white of the eyeball and the skin of the eyelid. Little red spots on the skin and bleeding while brushing teeth are signs of low platelets. Dehydration begins with dry mouth and sunken eyes. In severe cases there is "tenting" where skin that is pulled up will look like a tent after you let go. The best place to see the yellow color associated with jaundice is usually the conjunctiva of the eye or the frenulum, the tiny bit of tissue that connects the tongue to the bottom of the mouth.

Weight loss is a sign of poor nutrition. Is there *temporal wasting*? The temporalis muscle is a muscle that fills in an indentation on both sides of the skull—the temples at the sides of the forehead. This muscle is one of the last muscles that will become smaller in size when someone is not receiving enough nutrients. Patients who are very sick do not eat as much or as well, and cancer can diminish the body's ability to utilize nutrients appropriately.

What are other options besides the most aggressive therapy?

Besides aggressive treatment, there could be the option of chronic treatment, in which the treatment is designed to keep the cancer from spreading further but not eradicate it altogether. This therapy might be your first choice, or it might be a follow-up to aggressive treatment in cases where the cancer was not fully eradicated. If the tumor can be held in place, then this is called *stable disease*. In some cases, there are therapies that help to keep disease stable for a long time. Some of the new, targeted therapies will keep a tumor in check without entirely eliminating it. While doctors are still learning how to optimize treatment with targeted therapies, the current experiences are that these may work for a while and then a resistant group of cells emerges. But even this amount of time can be a wonderful gift to you.

What are alternative therapies?

These are therapies that are outside the standard medical treatments offered by the physician community. They may include mind and body treatments, such as yoga, and the more meditative martial arts such as tai chi. They may also include folk remedies, nutrition supplements, and over-the-counter drugs.

Can alternative therapies help me?

Certainly the immune system is boosted by relieving stress. However, if there has not been rigorous testing of a specific therapy in a clinical trial, then we can't really say that it will add to survival. It may add to your quality of life, though. If you believe in it, if it makes you feel good, and if it doesn't hurt you, then you should include alternative therapies in your personal treatment plan. However, you should let your doctor know what you are doing in addition to his or her treatment plan.

Can alternative therapies hurt me?

Yes, if anything that you are taking interferes with the medical therapy that you are receiving. It is important to let your medical oncologist, radiation oncologist, and surgeon know what supplements and over-the-counter drugs you are taking. Your diet may also play a factor in your response to therapy.

What if I do not want to receive any treatment, or any more treatment for my cancer?

There can be a period when palliative care is the right level of care. Palliative care is therapy to relieve pain and make you feel comfortable. Either a cancer was diagnosed after it had spread very far, or it has come back and metastasized. All the aggressive treatments have been tried, or you don't want to deal with the side-effects from the outset. Comfort and quality of life are the most important issues to you now. This can be a difficult decision, as much so for loved ones and caregivers as for the patients themselves. This is a time to hold hands and smile, and appreciate the sunrise and sunset on every day. It is a time to set up hospice care and to be pain-free. It might be tempting to be bitter; the parting gift resulting from your bitterness can be that your loved ones know you are unhappy and are relieved to see this unhappiness end for you. The downside is that their memories of you as a person will be affected by this period.

Choosing palliative care could also be a period of acceptance and long, lingering smiles. It is a time to put unanswered questions to rest and just let things be. When you make this decision, it is important to have a living will in place so that your wishes are properly followed.

How do I decide when palliative care is right for someone I love?

There is no straightforward formula for when palliative care becomes the appropriate solution. When you are around someone every day, it is sometimes hard to notice subtle changes that build up over time. There are some things that can be taken into account. How much weight has the patient lost? Does he or she have temporal wasting, where the muscles that usually fill in the space of the temples are getting smaller? When assessing how well someone is doing overall, doctors look for temporal wasting. It can be helpful as a sign that your loved one has become very, very weak, and that it may be a time to consider palliative care. If you are not sure, ask your doctor about it—is this a temporary thing that can be addressed or not?

Another sign is frequent bouts of minor infections that become serious rapidly. An example is frequent bladder infections that spread easily, leaving a patient confused and delirious. Low white cell counts, anemia, and low platelet count either from poor nutrition or interference by the cancer with the body's machinery to make these cells, can be indications that a cancer has recurred, or that it has progressed to a very aggressive state. Again, it is important to discuss your situation with your doctor to understand whether this is a reversible side-effect or not.

A very important thing to consider in this period if you choose palliative care or hospice care is relief of pain. No one should be afraid of becoming an addict at this time, and no one should be denied pain medication for this reason. To be pain-free is very important. Hospice care and the quality of care givers are also very important. A very useful resource can be the social worker in your hospital or an advocacy group that can help you identify a good organization that provides hospice care.

Where can I, as a caregiver or a patient, find a support group?

Both caregivers and patients undergo the challenge of stressful decisions as they endure difficult therapies during this time period. It can be a cause of great stress to accommodate both the emotional and physical level of care for a patient receiving any level of care, and perhaps one of the most difficult is palliative care. It is important to be able to access support, and to find advocates. I have added a Web site that lists a number of advocacy groups, many of which specifically address a certain type of tumors.

Also, check with your local treatment center for support services for patients and their caregivers. Give to yourself. Yoga, massage, relaxation, rest, and exercise all contribute to a tranquil state of mind and a healthy immune system. Larger cancer centers offer social services that not only help in identifying support groups, but they also help in deciphering insurance regulations. Cancer centers with SPORE awards include advocacy groups. Even if you cannot go to one of these cancer centers, a patient advocate might be able to help you find a support group for you that is closer to your home.

If you are having trouble finding an advocate or support group, or you need help in making your wishes known, ask for help from the Chief Nurse Administrator at the hospital where you are being cared for. There is generally a Chief Nurse Administrator on call around the clock. National advocacy groups such as the Live Strong Foundation might also be able to locate an advocacy group for you in your area.

Something very important is to remember the power of a smile. There is nothing so wonderful as smiling at someone and seeing them take in the moment and smile back.

Web sites to find hospitals that specialize in cancer treatment

http://www.cancer.gov/researchandfunding/extramural/cancercenters Maintained by the National Cancer Institute (NCI) and has information defining the cancer centers and a tool to find a cancer center near you. A list of NCI designated cancer centers and comprehensive cancer centers and their location can be found at this site http://www.cancer.gov/researchandfunding/extramural/cancercenters/find-a-cancer-center .

http://health.usnews.com/sections/health/ Maintained by the magazine *US News and World Report.* This site reviews cancer centers and ranks them according to their excellence (go to the Web site and either search for a link to the Best Hospital for Cancer or locate the link on the page for Best Hospital by Specialty and choose Cancer.

http://www.nccn.org/ Maintained by the National Cancer Center Network of cancer centers. The NCCN member cancer centers are listed under Patient Resources, or use the site search engine to search for Member Cancer Centers.

http://trp.cancer.gov/ A list of institutions that have a Specialized Program of Research Excellence (SPORE) grant awarded by the National Cancer Institute and focused on a specific type of cancer. Institutions with a SPORE award in, for example, breast cancer will have a large community of specialists dealing with breast cancer.

http://www.marycrowley.org A research foundation whose goal it is to make personalized therapy an option for every patient. They offer clinical trials that are focused on targeted therapies.

Web sites to find hospitals that specialize in cancer treatment, continued

http://www.aaci-cancer.org/ The official Web site for the American Association of Cancer Centers and whose mission is to promote the common interests of cancer centers. It maintains a membership directory. Cancer Centers can become members whether they have NCI designation or not.

Web sites for cancer statistics to learn how aggressive, or how indolent, your cancer is

http://seer.cancer.gov/ The Surveillance Epidemiology and End Results (SEER) published by the National Cancer Institute.

http://seer.cancer.gov/statistics/ Statistics in the Surveillance Epidemiology and End Results (SEER) published by the National Cancer Institute. Select the link to SEER Cancer Statistics Review for the years most recently reviewed and published (under the headline Annual reports and Monographs).

http://cancer.org Maintained by the American Cancer Society.

Websites to find advocacy and support groups for your cancer

http://www.cancertrialshelp.org/ An extensive list of patient advocacy groups is listed by the cooperative groups at their Web site. From this main page, go to the link titled "I am/I care for a patient with cancer" and, under the section titled Resources, go to Find a patient advocate.

Websites to find advocacy and support groups for your cancer, continued

http://trp.cancer.gov/ A list of institutions that have a Specialized Program of Research Excellence (SPORE) grant awarded by the National Cancer Institute and focused on a specific type of cancer. Institutions with a SPORE award in, for example, breast cancer will have a large community of specialists dealing with breast cancer. Each institution with a SPORE award maintains advocates for that cancer type.

http://www.cancer.gov/researchandfunding/extramural/can cercenters The web site has a tool to find a list of cancer centers and their locations, maintained by the National Cancer Institute. Cancer centers have patient advocacy and support groups.

Questions to ask your doctor

What types of therapy are you recommending for me-surgery, biological therapy, immunotherapy, targeted therapy, chemotherapy, and/or radiation therapy?

Why—please tell why for each type of therapy?

Should I get neo-adjuvant therapy—that is, therapy before surgery? What will I gain from it? What might I lose from it?

What are the chances that my tumor, if completely removed by surgery, will come back?

How will getting medical therapy or radiation keep that from happening?

What are the side-effects of the medical therapy or radiation?

Questions to ask your doctor, continued

If I need a second surgery—what will it accomplish? Is there a simpler way of doing it (e.g., laparoscopic surgery instead of major surgery)? What is a side-effect of the second surgery? Will I lose function? If I am willing to sacrifice that function, what are the chances that this surgery will cure me or give me longer to live?

How much longer? How many patients do you recommend having this surgery and how many are happy with the results?

For each type of therapy being recommended, and each type of agent (e.g., each chemotherapy drug), what are the benefits? How much of a chance of a cure can I expect? What are the side-effects? Which ones can be permanent? How often are they permanent?

Where can I get a second opinion?

Where can I find an advocacy or support group?

Where can my caregiver find resources for help?

Should I try to find a clinical trial for this diagnosis?

Chapter 8. What are clinical trials?

Terms included in this chapter (listed alphabetically)

Clinical trial
Phase I
Phase II
Phase III
Phase IV

What is a clinical trial?

A clinical trial is a research study either to find better ways to prevent a disease, to diagnose a disease, to make a prognosis for a patient, or to treat a disease. Clinical trials also have begun to address quality of life after treatment for a disease.

I will focus on clinical trials for cancer. These are divided into prevention trials, early detection or screening trials, diagnostic trials, quality of life or supportive-care trials, and treatment trials.

How do clinical trials come about?

Clinical treatment trials are initiated because a drug, a medical device, a treatment, or a procedure might have shown promise in animal or cell lines studies. Cell lines are lineages of cells that have been derived from cancer specimens and transformed so that they can be grown up in appropriate environments and will mimic the growth of the actual tumor.

Clinical trials for diagnosis and therapy are further classified as Phase I, Phase II, Phase III, or Phase IV trials. Each phase must be complete in order from I to IV before the next phase can begin.

What are Phase I clinical trials?

In Phase I trials, the safety of using the drug, device, procedure, etc., is tested. For a drug, this means trying it out at low doses to see what the side-effects are in humans. Phase I trials are not meant to test how effective a drug can be, and they might be performed at too low a dose to be effective.

What are Phase II clinical trials?

Phase II trials test the effectiveness of a new treatment in reducing cancer burden. The new drug or treatment is not compared to current modes of therapy—which would mean that it would be used alone in a subgroup of patients in the study—but is usually added to current therapy to see if it helps. Thus, typically patients in Phase II trials will also be receiving a standard regimen of therapy.

What are Phase III clinical trials?

In Phase III trials, a new regimen of therapy is compared to an existing regimen to decide which one is best. If the effect is small, then many, many patients are needed, and it may take years to evaluate the results. If the effect is larger, then fewer patients and typically less time are needed.

What is a Phase IV trial?

After a drug is licensed, then Phase IV trials (post marketing surveillance trials) monitor the wider use of the new medicine, looking at long-term survival and long-term side-effects.

How are the results of clinical trials evaluated?

Results from clinical trials are sent to biostatisticians to analyze. The data are often blinded, meaning that the statisticians do not know which patients are getting the new, test treatment and which are not. Trends are analyzed from early data so that if the results are strong enough early on, then new treatment plans will be offered to everyone. If there are sufficient adverse results, then the trial will be stopped to prevent bad outcomes from the test drug, device, or procedure.

Who joins clinical trials?

Some patients want to access trials so that they can be treated at the forefront of research. Other patients want a well-tried approach and have no interest in being in a trial. Yet others come in without a pre-formed opinion; and for others who have been through several treatments, a trial is the only option for treatment versus palliative care.

How do I find out if there is a clinical trial that I could join?

Clinical trials are sponsored by many different groups, including pharmaceutical companies; the National Cancer Institute; consortia of cancer centers called the Cooperative Groups that are geographically organized, e.g., the Southwest Oncology Group (SWOG); and other sources. Many oncologists in the community participate as affiliates in these trials, or communicate through cooperative groups to make trials available to their patients. Unfortunately, there is not one single Web site that a patient can go to in order to find a list of trials that he or she could join. However, there are a number of useful Web sites for finding trials, and these are given below in the Web site lists for this chapter.

Web sites for information on clinical trials

http://EmergingMed.com Maintained by an Internet information company that receives subscription fees from pharmaceutical and biotechnology companies to publish their trial information.

http://ClinicalTrials.gov Maintained by the National Library of Medicine, a sister institute to the National Cancer Institute. Both are institutes within the National Institute of Health.

Web sites for information on clinical trials, continued
http://www.cancer.gov/clinicaltrials/search/   A   search engine for trial information maintained by the National Cancer Institute

http://ResearchMatch.org A nonprofit Web site designed to match   up   patients   with   ongoing   clinical   trials. ResearchMatch is a Clinical and Translational Science Award   initiative   funded   by   the   National Center   for Research Resources,   a   sister   institute   to   the   National Cancer Institute. Both are institutes within the National Institute of Health.

http://CenterWatch.com   Maintained   by   an   Internet information company that receives subscription fees from pharmaceutical and biotechnology companies to publish their trial information.

http://SearchClinicalTrials.org   Maintained by a nonprofit organization called Center for Information and Study on Clinical Research Participation.

http://www.cancertrialshelp.org/   Maintained   by   the National   Cancer   Institute   Clinical   Trials   Cooperative Groups.

http://cancer.org maintained by the American Cancer Society.

http://www.nccn.org/clinical_trials/patients.asp Maintained by the National Cancer Center Network of cancer centers that are designated by the National Cancer Institute, and many of which are comprehensive cancer centers.

Web sites for information on clinical trials, continued
http://trp.cancer.gov   A list of institutions that have a Specialized Program of Research Excellence (SPORE) grant awarded by the National Cancer Institute and focused on a specific type of cancer. These research groups often have clinical trials in progress.

http://www.marycrowley.org A research foundation whose goal it is to make personalized therapy an option for every patient. They offer clinical trials that are focused on targeted therapies.

Questions to ask your doctor
Are there any clinical trials for my type of cancer?

Is this a phase I, II, III, or IV trial? Or a different type of trial (quality-of-life, etc.)?

How different will my therapy be from usual types of therapy?

What are my options and what would I get from this trial?

If this is a phase II or III trial, what did they learn from phase I—in other words, what will my side-effects be for this trial drug, device, or procedure?

How will my care be paid for in this clinical trial? What about any medications that I may receive?

Chapter 9. What happens if my cancer doesn't stay in remission?

> **Terms in this Chapter (listed alphabetically)**
> Recurrence
> Remission

What is remission?

At the beginning of cancer therapy, physicians tend to be the most aggressive in trying to eradicate the disease. If your cancer is treated and there is no evidence of it remaining, then you are in remission.

What happens after remission?

After a tumor goes into remission, patients are continually screened for a period of time. In general, during the first 5 years they have the closest screening. The 5-year period is somewhat arbitrary. When treatments were less effective, it was likely a more meaningful time interval at which to say you were cured. Now, we know that some cancers may still come back after longer than 5 years. The time interval depends on your cancer type. Some of this information is in the Surveillance Epidemiology and End Results tables or at the American Cancer Society Web site (see Web sites listed at the end of this chapter). Ask you doctor what the time interval is for your cancer beyond which there is very little likelihood of a recurrence.

What happens if you have a recurrence?

If there is a recurrence of the cancer, then the next step is typically to modify the therapy: add a new agent, either chemotherapy or radiation, or perform additional surgery. If all of the therapies are exhausted, patients are often encouraged to seek a clinical trial if they still want an aggressive therapy (see Chapters 7 and 8 and Web sites).

Over time, battling cancer can become a process of treating a chronic disease. This may continue with several successes over time, and new therapies may be introduced in an intervening period of remission. For example, in the last several years, several new clinical trials for kidney cancer have been introduced, in comparison to the previous decades where surgery was the only option. Treatment of melanoma is rapidly changing with the introduction of personalized therapies. Treatments of many other types of cancer are currently being addressed. A complete list is beyond the scope of this book. The important message is to know that new treatments may be available if you do recur.

How long should I go on treating recurrences?

When making a decision like this, be sure to think about quality of life. If you are sure that the next therapy will give you more time, and this is often very important for a parent of young children, then the chance of winning back more time seems more important than quality of life. But for someone else, quality of life will weigh in as more important. Each treatment will take another toll, and can this one be tolerated? Rethinking a course that might have started with aggressive therapy and switching over to palliative care is a decision that should take careful thought. Just as in making a treatment decision at the start of therapy, the same considerations discussed in Chapter 7 are important when treating a recurrence.

Why do tumors come back when we think they are completely gone?

We have learned over the last decade that tumor cells, once they escape from the primary tumor site, can circulate in our bloodstream. They may not have the ability to thrive in foreign tissues, so they might slowly disappear, or they might hide out someplace in a state of stasis. They may never return from stasis, or they might acquire the capability of growing in foreign territory. It may also be that, over time, your own immune system that has been keeping them in check is no longer working as well.

Useful websites for cancer statistics

http://seer.cancer.gov/ The Surveillance Epidemiology and End Results published by the National Cancer Institute.

http://seer.cancer.gov/statistics/ Statistics in the Surveillance Epidemiology and End Results published by the National Cancer Institute. Select the link to SEER Cancer Statistics Review for the years most recently reviewed and published (under the headline Annual Reports and Monographs).

http://cancer.org Maintained by the American Cancer Society.

Questions for your doctor

Am I in remission?

How long will I likely stay in remission?

After how long will there be little likelihood that I will have a recurrence?

What should my cancer surveillance plan be now, and after 5 years following my first diagnosis?

Chapter 10. How can I donate my cancer tissue for research?

Terms used in this chapter (listed alphabetically)
Background information
Follow-up information
HIPAA
Intellectual property
Security
Tissue donation
45CFR46

Human tissue samples are vital to the development of new medical therapies, especially those based on targeting specific molecules in a cancer cell. It is important not only to have the tissue for research, but to also have the background information and the follow-up information. Background information is the information about you before you were diagnosed with cancer, and follow-up information is the information about you after you were diagnosed with cancer. To consent to donate tissue, and added to that to consent to allow your background and follow-up information to be attached to the tissue, are wonderful gifts to others as long as your privacy is appropriately protected as specified by local, state, and federal regulations. The use of your tissue and follow-up information along with the protection of your identity are covered by certain laws and regulations set up to protect your privacy. These will be described below.

Who oversees how tissue is used for research?

Use of tissue and associated information in research is governed at the federal, state, and local level by laws that govern protection of human subjects being used for research. At the federal level, human subjects research protection is regulated by the Code of Federal Regulations Title 45, Part 46 (45CFR46) and by the Health Insurance Portability and Accountability Act (HIPAA). Many states have passed legislation governing use of tissue and information. At the local level there is a board that reviews procedures for collection of tissue and clinical information. This group is usually called the Institutional Review Board (IRB) or the Institutional Ethics Committee (IEC) at the local level, and it must be registered with the Office for Human Research Protection (OHRP) if the research is conducted or supported by any agency of the U.S. Department of Health and Human Services (HHS). Members of an IRB or IEC may include local religious leaders, physician/scientists, and ethicists.

How is my privacy protected?

Your privacy is covered under 45CFR46 and HIPAA. Under 45CFR46, one provision for using your tissue and information for research is that if the tissue and information is completely stripped of your identifiers and there is no way to link them back to your record, then it is acceptable to distribute them for research. This can be done without your consent, although most local review boards will specify that if a patient refuses to donate tissue, then it cannot be distributed for research even if it is completely stripped of identifiers. This means that at the time that the tissue and information is given to a researcher, all subsequent follow-up information will not be available to the researcher because the link back to your record is permanently broken. This limits the ability of the researcher to link properties of the cancer to how you might have responded to therapy, whether you had a recurrence, and how long your survival is. Some research does not require this information. However, in general, the tissue is more valuable to research into medical therapy if continuing follow-up information is available.

This rule also means that once the pathologist has taken the tissue he or she needs to make a diagnosis, the rest of the tissue from your surgery, called remnant tissue, can be permanently de-identified or anonymized and distributed for research without your consent. If the hospital where you have surgery collects remnant tissue for research, you may want to make sure that it is truly permanently stripped of its identifiers before it is released.

There is another scenario acceptable to 45CFR46 for use of human tissue and information in research. In this case, an "honest broker" model is used to distribute tissue and information for research.

What is an "honest broker" model?

If tissue and information is collected and coded, and a key to decipher the code is not distributed to the researcher, then the de-identified tissue and information can be released. This allows the researcher to go back to the person who distributed the tissue and information with the code associated with your tissue, and ask for more information. The distributor is the *honest broker*, who will go into the files, link the code to your identifier, abstract more information, scrub it of any identifying details, and distribute it to the researcher. These files that link the code to your identifier cannot be released by the honest broker, and the honest broker cannot be directly involved in the research.

So does this mean that my consent is not required for tissue and information to be released to researchers?

Yes, it is technically not required if the information is stripped of all of your identifiers, or if the local IRB or IEC accepts a working honest broker system. But, it is up to the local IRB or IEC to make that decision. Some IRBs and IECs will still require that you sign an informed consent even though it is not technically required by 45CFR46. In addition, whether or not your consent is required, the local IRB or IEC reviews the research protocols to make sure that they are ethical and that your privacy is protected.

The situation is more complex if the research is carried out under the auspices of the hospital, which is a "covered entity" under HIPAA. The rules of HIPAA require that a covered entity keep a log of whoever has access to your information, and that you have consented to its use. So a research organization that is not covered by HIPAA has only to be compliant with 45CFR46, but a hospital that performs research has to be compliant with both 45CFR46 and HIPAA. Under these circumstances, the local IRB and IEC groups will typically require your consent for use of any tissue.

Should I have any concerns about how my privacy is protected?

The honest broker model and the use of tissue and information with informed consent can all work to protect your information as long as your identifiers are stored in a secure place that is not accessible to those who should not access it. If you want to donate tissue and information for research, and the hospital where you are having surgery has the facilities to collect such tissue, then you can ask it about its IRB or IEC, whether it uses an honest broker model or it requires informed consent, and whether it secures the computer systems and files where your identity is stored. The hospital should protect it behind a firewall (or locked file in a private, locked office if it is on paper) that restricts access to the information. If it is stored in a computer system, then access should also be controlled by a login procedure that requires an identifier and password. Since many hospitals use secured computers to store your clinical charts in an electronic medical record system, then they are well-versed in the security systems required to protect your identifiers.

Can I refuse to have my tissue used?

Most hospitals will respect your right to refuse to have tissue used, even if it is completely stripped of identifiers as regulated by 45CFR46. If this is your desire, speak to your doctor or surgeon about your wishes. If you have difficulty finding someone to help you, there is a Chief Nurse Administrator at most if not all hospitals whom you can call upon for help in resolving this issue.

If I sign a consent for my tissue to be used, can I revoke it later?

You have the right to revoke your consent. Most IRBs and IECs require that there is a procedure in place for retrieving any tissue or information that has not been distributed for which consent has been revoked, and removing it from the inventory of tissue and information that is accessible for research.

Is donating my tissue and information for research a good thing to do?

As I stated at the beginning of the chapter, tissue donation is vital to making progress in treating cancer. We are looking forward to the day when medical treatment is personalized, when we can identify any unique properties of a cancer that will affect how the patient is treated. We can only learn the unique and personal characteristics of cancer by studying cancer tissue donated by patients, and studying its genes and proteins in relation to the patient's health and response to therapy. When the hospital has in place appropriate security for your privacy and oversees ethical use of tissue in research, then donating your tissue and information is a great gift to future patients with cancer. However, this is a personal decision for each patient. You are within your rights to refuse consent if you have any privacy concerns or any personal reasons that would prohibit you from donating tissue.

If a discovery is made from the tissue, will I receive any compensation for it?

No, and there have been court cases that address this issue. Since the intellectual contributions were made by the investigators who used your tissue in research, then the results are the intellectual property of the institution and the investigators, according to whatever policy the institution has in place for sharing intellectual property with the investigator.

Does my tissue and information belong to the investigator or group of investigators that collected and are using it, or to the institution where it was collected?

The tissue and patient information belongs to the institution. It is the institution that provides the infrastructure necessary to collect, store, and distribute this tissue, and that provides the oversight for its ethical use. If an investigator moves to another institution, he or she cannot take a tissue collection with them. In general, discoveries made today rely upon a team approach. Tissue-based research involves special preparation methods for the tissues, expensive and complex technologies to study them, and many investigators and statisticians to interpret the results. To give the full team credit, the institution takes ownership of the tissue, and also takes responsibility for insuring its ethical use and the protection of the donors' privacy.

Will genetic information about me be discovered that can harm me?

Genetic information about you might be discovered. Some of it may be somatic, so it should not affect you or your family members in the way that germline genetic information can. It is the role of the IRB and the IEC of the local institution to set up barriers to any of this information being used against you, and also to protect your privacy. The newly passed Genetic Information Nondiscrimination Act (GINA) of 2008 is designed to protect you. This new federal law protects us from being discriminated against by health insurers and by employers because of our genetic make-up. Some legal experts have questioned how difficult it might be to apply the law though. When giving tissue for research, the most important protection in place is the security of the data that is collected and the protection of your identity.

Web sites with information on regulations concerning human research protections and protection from discrimination based on genetic information

http://www.hhs.gov/ohrp/humansubjects/guidance/ For information on 45CFR 46. Answers to FAQs are at http://answers.hhs.gov/ohrp/categories/1562

http://www.hhs.gov/ocr/hipaa/ For information on HIPAA.

http://www.genome.gov/10002328#3 For the fact sheet about the Genetic Information Nondiscrimination Act (GINA) of 2008.

Questions for your doctor

Can I donate tissue for research?

Do I need to sign an informed consent form?

Who will access my information?

How is my privacy protected?

Who will oversee the ethical use of my tissue?

Who will benefit?

Chapter 11. What's on the horizon in cancer medicine?

At this point in medicine, we feel poised at the exciting verge of seeing a tremendous change in how cancer is managed. We look forward to a time when each patient's tumor will be carefully screened and a battery of drugs are applied that are known to work well on the specific types of tumor cells that a patient has. Cancer cells are targeted, much like the "Death Star" in the first *Star Wars* movie (*Episode IV*). One thing we have learned is our tumors are not like a simple Death Star that has one weak site, but more like a Death Stars with multiple key sites that need to be removed. (What would Darth Vader say to hear his Death Star called simple?) It is likely that in the future patients will be receiving multiple therapies, each targeted at a single molecule working separately or in a network. We are beginning to make progress in getting there with the epidermal growth factor receptor therapies, the anti-angiogenesis therapies, the anti-Her2/neu therapies, several new kidney cancer therapies, new melanoma therapies, and targeted therapy for gastrointestinal stromal tumors. If you are diagnosed with a tumor, try to research developments in targeted therapies for that tumor and see what is happening. There might be a clinical trial. And, if not now, there may be one in time for a recurrence.

In addition to these molecularly targeted therapies, vaccines for cancer, or to prevent causes of cancer, are being added to treatment options today. The development of a vaccine to prevent viral infections that can cause cervical cancer is an important new development. This is a prevention vaccine. But, it is also important to know that the vaccine currently available does not prevent all types of human papilloma virus (HPV) that cause cervical cancer, in addition to the fact that most but *not* all of cervical cancers are caused by HPV.

There are also vaccines that attack tumor cells. These are vaccines that take substances from your tumor and present them to your immune system so that your immune system will reject your tumor. Vaccine therapy for melanoma has demonstrated remarkable results for many patients. Vaccines are also being developed to treat other cancers.

As these targeted therapies become more specific to someone's cancer, i.e., "personalized therapy," it becomes increasingly important to be able to know the identifying characteristics of a tumor that make it susceptible to targeted therapy. If a small subset of patients with lung cancer respond remarkably to a drug, but the number is so small that it is swamped by the number of patients who receive no benefit from it, then a clinical trial that includes all lung cancer patients may not prove its benefit. However, if we know which tumors will be responsive, the clinical trial can be focused on the patients who have responsive tumors. Even as we develop new drugs, we are not always sure which patients they are best suited to. This is one of the reasons why donating tissue for research can benefit the cancer patient community.

Trying to summarize all of the available targeted therapies available even now would be like trying to hit a moving target. Some are available as standard therapy while others are still in clinical trials. Many if not all major cancer centers offer clinical trials using personalized approaches (see Web sites for Clinical Trials at the end of Chapter 8, and the List of Useful Web sites at the end of this book). Notably, President Barack Obama, when he was a Senator, introduced the Genomics and Personalized Medicine Act in 2007 to secure the promise of personalized medicine by expanding and accelerating genomics research, to support initiatives to improve the accuracy of disease diagnosis, and to increase the safety of drugs while identifying novel treatments. While the bill did not reach the Senate floor, the message here is that there is *much* interest at the national level in developing personalized medicine.

List of useful Web sites

Web sites for cancer statistics

http://seer.cancer.gov/ The Surveillance Epidemiology and End Results published, by the National Cancer Institute. Select the "Cancer Statistics" tab (or go directly there by going to http://seer.cancer.gov/statistics). You can either select "Fast Stats" to access the statistics organized by organ site, ethnicity, gender, and other variables, or for more detailed information about the SEER statistics select "Cancer Statistics Review". By selecting the "Publications" tab, you can access the link to "Monographs" and select the latest "SEER Survival Monograph" for perusal.

Web sites for cancer statistics to learn how aggressive, or how indolent, your cancer is

http://seer.cancer.gov/ The Surveillance Epidemiology and End Results (SEER) published by the National Cancer Institute.

http://seer.cancer.gov/statistics/ Statistics in the Surveillance Epidemiology and End Results (SEER) published by the National Cancer Institute. Select the link to SEER Cancer Statistics Review for the years most recently reviewed and published (under the headline Annual reports and Monographs).

http://cancer.org Maintained by the American Cancer Society.

Web sites for information about genetic testing

http://www.nsgc.org/ is a Web site maintained by the National Society of Genetic Counselors. They provide a link for finding a genetic counselor near you.

Web sites for information about genetic testing, continued.

http://www.genome.gov/10002328#3 is a Web site maintained by the National Human Genome Research Institute (NHGRI). It has a fact sheet about the Genetic Information Nondiscrimination Act (GINA) of 2008

http://www.genome.gov is the web site for the home page of the National Human Genome Research Institute (NHGRI) Web site. It contains general information about the state of research into human genetics

---

Web sites for information on screening recommendations.

http://www.cancer.org Maintained by the American Cancer Society. Go to this Web site and search for screening or early detection.

http://cdc.gov Maintained by the Centers for Disease Control and Prevention. Go to this Web site and search for preventive cancer screening.

http://cancer.gov Maintained by the National Cancer Institute. Go to this Web site, scroll down to Cancer Topics, and click on the link to *Screening And Testing.*

Web sites for current research and clinical trials to screen for a specific type of cancer

http://cancer.gov Maintained by the National Cancer Institute with listings by cancer type. For example, for lung cancer screening trials go to http://cancer.gov, scroll down to Cancer Topics, click on the link to *Screening And Tests*, and then click on the link to *Lung Cancer: Screening And Testing.* Scroll down and look for a link to clinical trials for screening tests under study.

Web site with general information about sentinel lymph node biopsy

http://www.cancer.gov/cancertopics/factsheet/Therapy/sentinel-node-biopsy This Web site is created by the National Cancer Institute.

Web sites to find a place to seek a second opinion or to find a hospital that specializes in cancer

http://www.cancer.gov/researchandfunding/extramural/cancercenters Maintained by the National Cancer Institute (NCI) and has information defining the cancer centers and a tool to find a cancer center near you. A list of NCI designated cancer centers and comprehensive cancer centers and their location can be found at this site http://www.cancer.gov/researchandfunding/extramural/cancercenters/find-a-cancer-center .

http://health.usnews.com/sections/health/ Maintained by the magazine *US News and World Report.* This site reviews cancer centers and ranks them according to their excellence (go to the Web site and either search for a link to the Best Hospital for Cancer or locate the link on the page for Best Hospital by Specialty and choose Cancer.

http://www.nccn.org/ Maintained by the National Cancer Center Network of cancer centers. The NCCN member cancer centers are listed under Patient Resources, or use the site search engine to search for Member Cancer Centers.

http://trp.cancer.gov/ A list of institutions that have a Specialized Program of Research Excellence (SPORE) grant awarded by the National Cancer Institute and focused on a specific type of cancer. Institutions with a SPORE award in, for example, breast cancer will have a large community of specialists dealing with breast cancer.

Web sites to find a place to seek a second opinion or to find a hospital that specializes in cancer, continued

http://www.aaci-cancer.org/ The official Web site for the American Association of Cancer Centers and whose mission is to promote the common interests of cancer centers. It maintains a membership directory. Cancer Centers can become members whether they have NCI designation or not.

http://www.marycrowley.org A research foundation whose goal it is to make personalized therapy an option for every patient. They offer clinical trials that are focused on targeted therapies.

Web sites for information on clinical trials in general

http://EmergingMed.com Maintained by an Internet information company that receives subscription fees from pharmaceutical and biotechnology companies to publish their trial information.

http://ClinicalTrials.gov Maintained by the National Library of Medicine, a sister institute to the National Cancer Institute. Both are institutes within the National Institute of Health.

http://www.cancer.gov/clinicaltrials/search/ A search engine for trial information maintained by the National Cancer Institute

http://ResearchMatch.org A nonprofit Web site designed to match up patients with ongoing clinical trials. ResearchMatch is a Clinical and Translational Science Award initiative funded by the National Center for Research Resources, a sister institute to the National Cancer Institute. Both are institutes within the National Institute of Health.

Web sites for information on clinical trials in general, continued

http://CenterWatch.com Maintained by an Internet information company that receives subscription fees from pharmaceutical and biotechnology companies to publish their trial information.

http://SearchClinicalTrials.org Maintained by a nonprofit organization called Center for Information and Study on Clinical Research Participation.

http://www.cancertrialshelp.org/ Maintained by the National Cancer Institute Clinical Trials Cooperative Groups.

http://Cancer.org maintained by the American Cancer Society.

http://www.nccn.org/clinical_trials/patients.asp Maintained by the National Cancer Center Network of cancer centers that are designated by the National Cancer Institute, and many of which are comprehensive cancer centers.

http://trp.cancer.gov/ A list of institutions that have a Specialized Program of Research Excellence (SPORE) grant awarded by the National Cancer Institute and focused on a specific type of cancer. These research groups often have clinical trials in progress.

http://www.marycrowley.org A research foundation whose goal it is to make personalized therapy an option for every patient. They offer clinical trials that are focused on targeted therapies.

Websites to find advocacy and support groups for your cancer

http://www.cancertrialshelp.org/ An extensive list of patient advocacy groups is listed by the cooperative groups at their Web site. From this main page, go to the link titled "I am/I care for a patient with cancer" and, under the section titled Resources, go to Find a patient advocate.

http://trp.cancer.gov/ A list of institutions that have a Specialized Program of Research Excellence (SPORE) grant awarded by the National Cancer Institute and focused on a specific type of cancer. Institutions with a SPORE award in, for example, breast cancer will have a large community of specialists dealing with breast cancer. Each institution with a SPORE award maintains advocates for that cancer type.

http://www.cancer.gov/researchandfunding/extramural/cancercenters The web site has a tool to find a list of cancer centers and their locations, maintained by the National Cancer Institute. Cancer centers have patient advocacy and support groups.

Web sites with information on regulations concerning human research protections and protection from discrimination based on genetic information

http://www.hhs.gov/ohrp/humansubjects/guidance/ For information on 45CFR 46. Answers to FAQs are at http://answers.hhs.gov/ohrp/categories/1562

http://www.hhs.gov/ocr/hipaa/ For information on HIPAA.

http://www.genome.gov/10002328#3 For the fact sheet about the Genetic Information Nondiscrimination Act (GINA) of 2008.

Index

101

102

Made in the USA
San Bernardino, CA
30 March 2017